VEGAN KETO COOKBOOK

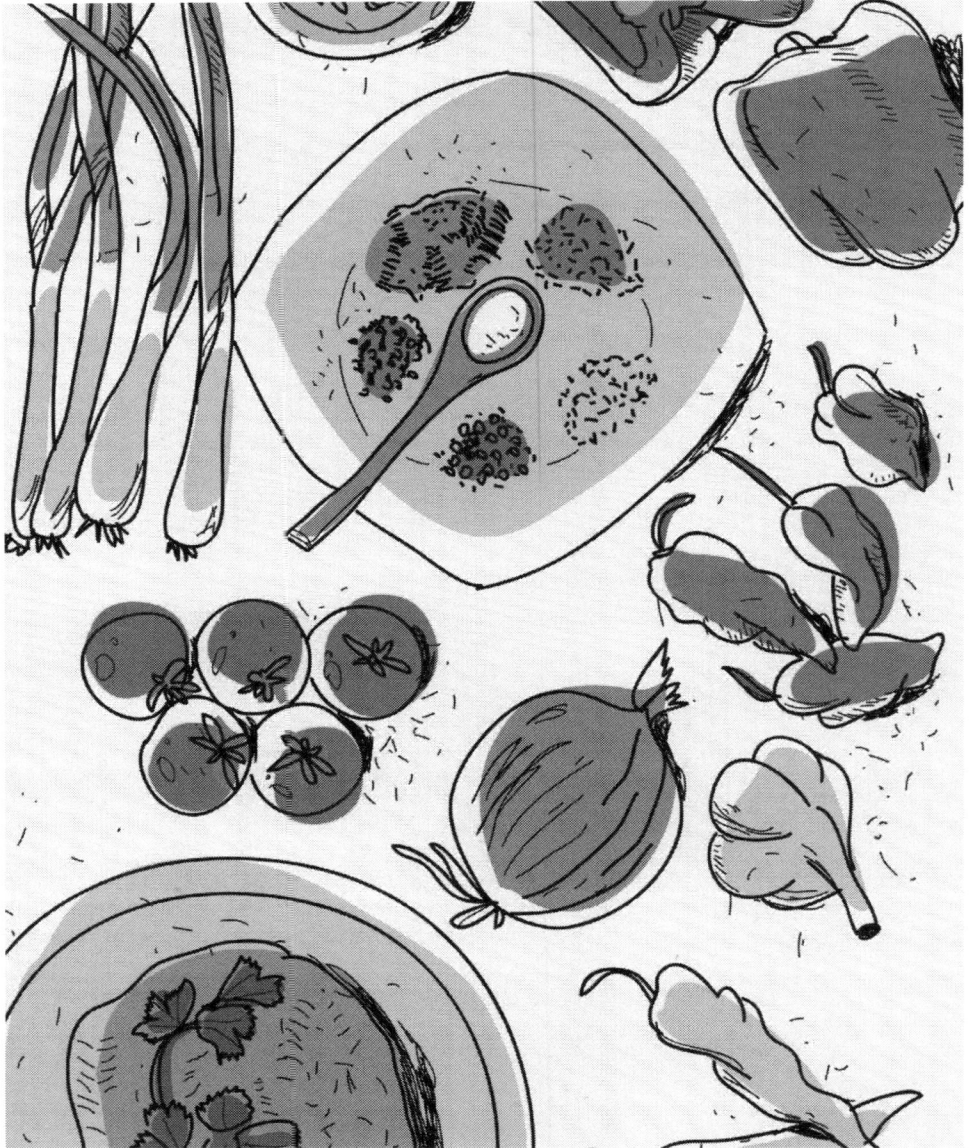

VEGAN
KETO
Cookbook

30 Day Meal Plan and 100 Vegan Ketogenic Diet Recipes for Enjoying A Low-Carb Plant-Based Vegan Keto Lifestyle

Elli Thomston

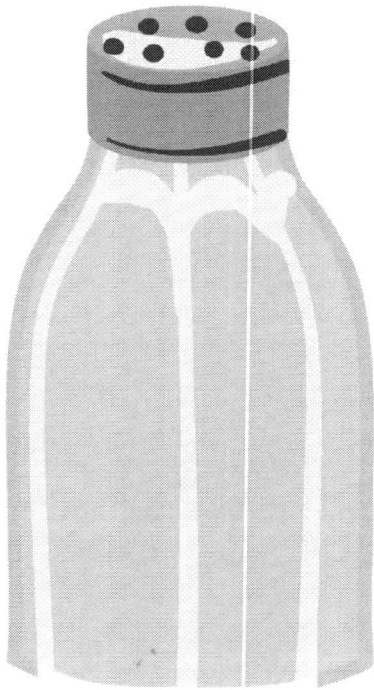 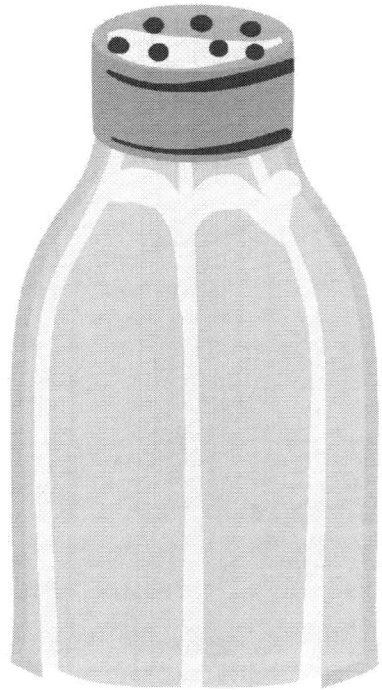

4

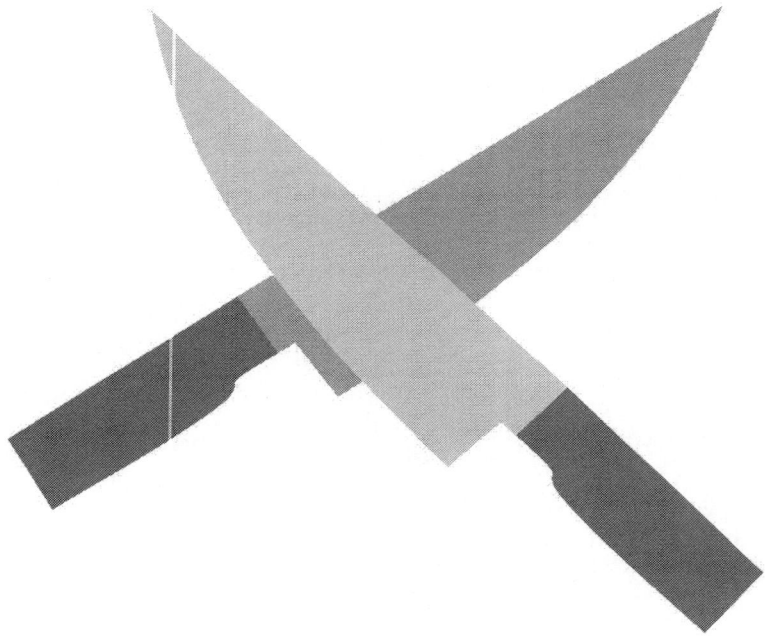

CONTENTS

FORWARD 9

HOW I WENT KETO AS A VEGAN 11

I. INTRODUCTION TO THE KETOGENIC AND VEGAN DIETS 12

II. COMBINING THE KETOGENIC DIET WITH THE VEGAN DIET 17

III. EVERYTHING YOU NEED TO KNOW TO SUCCEED ON THE KETOGENIC VEGAN DIET .. 23

BREAKFAST RECIPES 27

SOUPS AND SALADS RECIPES 49

SNACKS AND SIDES RECIPES 71

LUNCH RECIPES 89

DINNER RECIPES 107

DESSERT RECIPES 125

REFERENCES AND RESOURCES 142

THE "DIRTY DOZEN" AND "CLEAN 15" 145

MEASUREMENT CONVERSION TABLES 147

INDEX 148

30 DAY MEAL PLAN 150

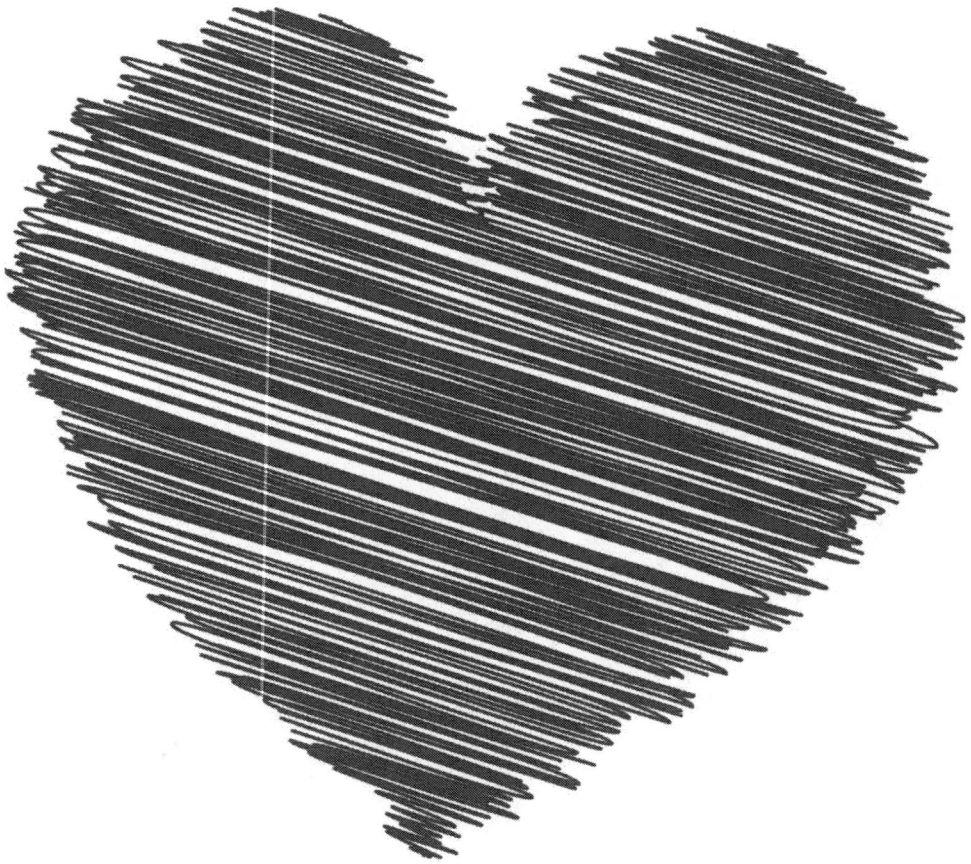

FORWARD

Hippocrates' patient had a problem. He suffered from seizures and didn't know what to do to stop them. Hippocrates recommended fasting. During the days the patient didn't eat or drink, he was seizure-free! Why did it work? In the centuries since the time of Hippocrates, doctors have learned about ketones, anticonvulsant compounds produced by the liver, that form when you don't eat. They also appear when you cut down on your carb intake and increase your intake of the fat found in coconuts, avocados, and other foods. This high-fat, low-carb diet has become known as the ketogenic diet and it comes with a variety of benefits, including improved energy levels, increased concentration, and easier weight loss.

For centuries, people have refrained from eating animals for all kinds of reasons, including religious ones. In 1944, the term "veganism" was first used to describe vegetarianisms who didn't consume *any* animals products, including dairy. This diet grows in popularity every year as we learn more about the effects of meat and the treatment of animals. The benefits of a strict plant-based diet include healthier skin and possibly protection from a variety of serious illnesses. Vegans who are fully invested in an animal-free life will even refuse to wear leather or feathers.

Both the ketogenic and vegan diets have long histories, and many people are beginning to combine them. Why? They can fill in each other's nutritional gaps and boost some of the benefits, including increased energy and reduced inflammation. It is a challenging (and for some complicated) diet that cuts out meat, dairy, grains, sugar, and foods high in carbs. In this book, we've organized all the information into easy-to-understand sections and lists for food, supplements, and electrolytes, so you can do this diet the healthy way. You'll learn why it's worth it and how it applies to your life when you hit the recipe section, which includes breakfasts, lunches, dinners, and desserts.

Whether you've been on the keto or vegan diet by themselves, or you're starting from scratch, this book will help guide you on everything you need to know about the science to the diet's drawbacks to what to expect during the first few weeks.

Sincerely,

Alex Gant

Diet Researcher

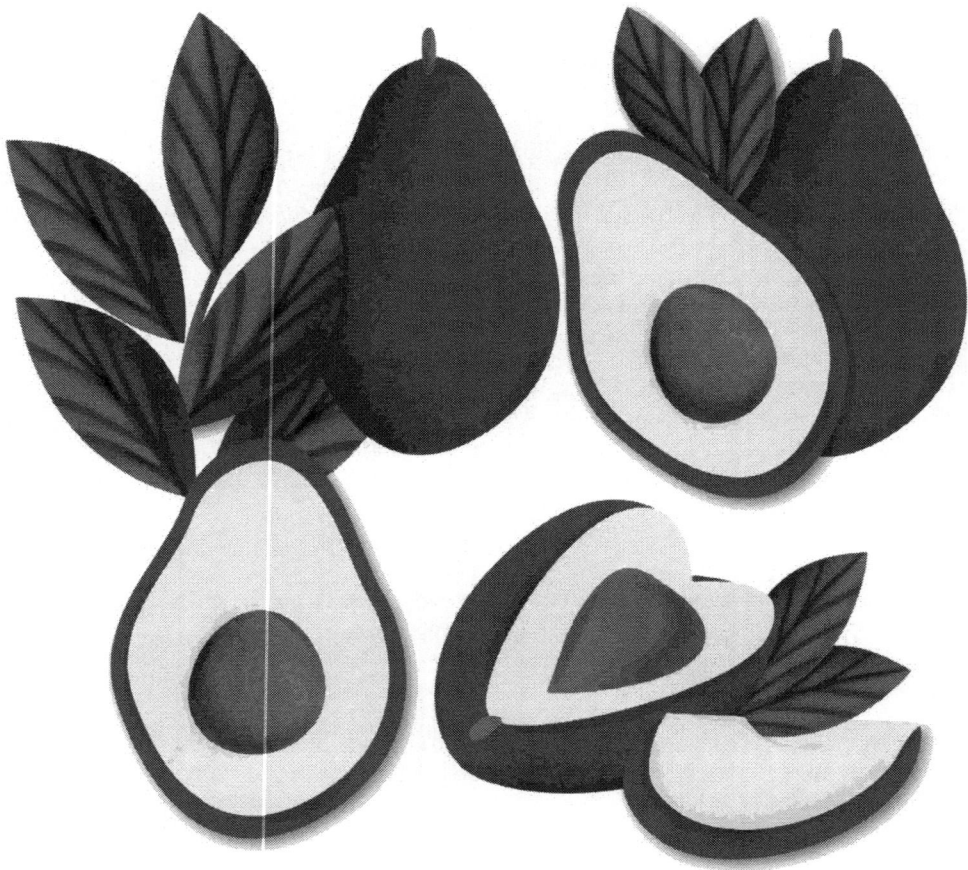

HOW I WENT KETO AS A VEGAN

When people start the vegan ketogenic diet, they've often already been eating keto or vegan. Not me. I started completely from scratch, and this book represents everything I learned over the last decade, or wished I would have known beforehand.

I first heard about the vegan diet since it's been popular among celebrities, athletes, and health nuts alike for a long time. The ketogenic diet, though it's been around just as long and has origins in ancient times, has only somewhat recently become mainstream. In the past, it was followed mostly by epileptics to ease their seizures. Now, it seems like everyone is singing the praises of bulletproof coffee and keto snack bars. I considered just going keto for a while, but when I started doing more research, I wasn't convinced it went quite far enough for me.

You see, I've never been a fan of the meat industry; I even experimented with being a vegetarian in college when I couldn't afford meat. My body also doesn't do well with dairy, so the full-fat dairy requirements of the keto diet weren't ideal. Then I started reading about vegans who were "going keto" and focusing on the fats found in plant-based foods. I didn't even know it was possible to hit ketosis without meat and dairy! Knowing that it was, I decided to make the big transition.

It wasn't easy. There's a lot I wish I knew beforehand, and I've included it all in the book. I wish I knew just how important tracking my electrolytes would be during the first few weeks, and that supplements are an important part of the diet right alongside the right foods. From what I've read and heard from people who were either vegan or keto beforehand, it's easier to make the transition if you're already in ketosis, at least from a physical standpoint. Mentally, it's obviously hard to give up meat and cheese, but the process of ketosis can cause flu-like symptoms if your diet was previously heavy in carbs.

> To stick to the ketogenic vegan diet, there are five things I had to remember:
> #1: No animal products
> #2: No grains
> #3: Eat only 20 grams of net carbs every day
> #4: Eat between 0.4-0.6 grams of protein per pound of your body weight every day
> #5: Get tested for nutrient lows and take supplements if needed

I also found that being really intentional about where I was getting my fat and keeping a food diary helped immensely. Now that I've been on the diet for many years, I can honestly say I've never felt better. I have more energy, I'm sleeping better, my mind is sharper, and I'm happier. My hope is that you experience positive changes in your life, as well, as a result of this book and the ketogenic vegan diet.

Yours in good health,

Elli Thomston

I. INTRODUCTION TO THE KETOGENIC AND VEGAN DIETS

These days, it seems like everyone is on some kind of new diet. People are going keto or going vegan, but what does that actually mean? Both the ketogenic (known as the keto diet for short) and vegan diets have been around for a long time, but are gaining in popularity as people move away from processed food, carbs, meat, and dairy. This section breaks down both diets, how they work, and what you can eat.

THE KETOGENIC DIET

In ancient times, doctors realized that refraining from food stopped people from having seizures. Fasting became the go-to treatment for epilepsy for centuries until physicians finally developed a diet that could mimic its effects. In 1921, a physician discovered that the liver produced three water-soluble compounds - which are called ketones - when a patient fasted *or* when they ate a diet high in fat and low in carbs. After a Mayo Clinic doctor conducted more research, the ketogenic diet was created. It then replaced fasting as the most popular treatment for epilepsy and in the 1990's, it went through a sort of Renaissance and people began adopting it for other health benefits. We'll discuss those a bit later, but first, let's explore what's going on in the body when you eat a lot of fat and cut down on carbs.

Using fat instead of carbs for fuel

Most people eat a lot of carbs, and while the body actually needs carbs to flourish, most of us eat too many. The body transforms carbs into glucose for fuel, but the excess gets stored as body fat. When you significantly cut down the amount of carbs you eat and replace it with fat, the body is forced to rely on fat for fuel. Now, the body can't actually use fat; it has to break the acids down first, and during this process, ketones are produced. These compounds are also used for fuel and are especially effective for the brain, your muscles, and mitochondria. The best part? Any ketones that aren't used are expelled through waste instead of stored as body fat.

To trigger "ketosis," the process of ketone production, you need to eat a specific ratio of fat, carbs, and protein. During the development of the ketogenic diet, doctors figured out that ketosis begins when your daily calorie count consists of 60-75% fat, 5-10% carbs, and the rest from protein. That translates into about 20 net carbs per day. You get net carbs by subtracting fiber from your total carbs, because fiber carbs don't count. To save time, you can learn how many grams of fat and protein you should eat using online calculators that also factor in your weight, weight goal, activity level, and so on.

How do you know when you're in ketosis?

You're following the ketogenic diet and sticking to your ratios, but how do you know if it's working? You can actually test your ketone level with urine strips, blood tests, or breath analyzers. Urine strips are cheap and best when you're first starting on the diet, because your body loses more ketones. The next method, blood tests, cost a bit more, but they're also more accurate. Breath tests are the priciest, though you just need to buy it once. The longer you're on the diet, the more ketones your body actually uses, so your test results will be lower.

Most tests measure ketones in mmol/L, or millimoles per liter. You'll be in ketosis when your result is anywhere between 1.5 and 3.0 mmol/L. If you're diabetic, you actually want to max out at just 1.5, because ketones make the blood more acidic, and acidic blood (known as ketoacidosis) can be life-threatening.

> **The ketogenic diet gets its name from and is based on the process of ketosis ,which is when the liver begins to produce chemical compounds known as ketones and the body relies on fat for fuel. To enter ketosis, you must eat a certain percentage of fat, protein, and carbs.**

Benefits of the keto diet

The ketogenic diet's ability to prevent seizures has been well-known for decades, but in the last few years, the diet has really taken off for people who don't have epilepsy. This is because of additional health benefits, such as:

Easier weight loss

When you stick to the keto diet, you eliminate a lot of foods that cause weight gain. The most significant elimination is sugar in all its forms, even natural sugars. Many studies show that sugar, not fat, is what causes weight gain, so when you cut it out of your diet, you might find that losing weight is much easier.

Higher energy levels

Carbs, especially the refined carbs you find in white bread, white rice, and so on, have a sleepy effect on the body. When you eat too many, that excess glucose spikes your blood sugar, giving you a temporary energy burst, which is then followed by an inevitable crash. When you replace most carbs with fat, your energy level might increase because your blood sugar levels are more stable. You won't go through carb rushes and crashes throughout your day.

Sharper cognitive functions

The brain loves using fat as fuel, and the keto diet is packed with food rich in brain-healthy fats. Consuming these while cutting out carbs can result in less "brain fog" and increased concentration. Many people find they're able to work, read, and focus for longer periods of time without feeling scattered. In fact, early research suggests the keto diet might help treat Alzheimer's, since higher ketone levels are linked to better memory retention.

Reduced pain

Many people suffer from aching joints, which is caused by inflammation. It can make exercise difficult, and even just sitting for long periods of time can cause pain. Inflammation can also cause problems like headaches and chronic fatigue. Sugar is a major cause of inflammation, so when you're on the keto diet and cutting it out, your body has a chance to heal. Arthritic pain and other symptoms are reduced significantly, allowing you to live your life.

The keto diet food list

What you can eat on the keto diet is determined by its carb content. Anything that's low-glycemic and doesn't have a huge effect on your blood sugar is acceptable, because it will keep you in ketosis. Anything that's high-glycemic and *does* affect your blood sugar a lot kicks you out of ketosis, so those are not allowed. The best keto foods will be high in fat and other nutrients, while low in carbs.

What you can eat:

- Full-fat dairy (except cow's milk)
- Grass-fed and pasture-raised meat (beef, chicken, pork, lamb, etc)
- Wild-caught seafood (fish, shellfish, etc)
- Eggs
- Low-glycemic vegetables (dark leafy greens, tomatoes, bell peppers, etc)
- Low-glycemic fruit (berries, avocados, lemons, limes, oranges)
- Nuts/seeds (macadamia nuts, almonds, cashews, pecans, etc)
- Healthy fats and oils (EVOO, coconut oil, nut butters, etc)

What you can't eat:

- All grains (pasta, bread, cereal, etc)
- Packaged, processed foods
- Low-fat, "diet" foods
- High-glycemic vegetables (potatoes, root vegetables)
- High-glycemic fruit (bananas, apples, most fruit)
- Refined sugar (ice cream, chocolate, candy, soda pop, etc)
- Refined oils (corn oil, vegetable oil, grapeseed oil, etc)

THE VEGAN DIET

Vegetarianism has existed in many civilizations for centuries. Some people also refused to consume any animal products, but it wasn't until 1944 that the philosophy got an official name. After members of the Vegetarian Society had their request for a newsletter section dedicated to non-dairy vegetarianism turned down, Donald Watson began his own publication. He named it "The Vegan News," combining the first three and last two letters of "vegetarian."

Not long after, a Vegan Society was formed. The founder of its British incarnation, Leslie J. Cross, defined veganism as seeking "an end to the use of animals by man for food, commodities, work, hunting, vivisection, and by all other uses involving exploitation of animal life by man." Today, you can find "ethical" vegans sticking to this rigid standard that not only entails a refusal to eat animal products, but also a dedication to not wearing or using them in any form.

Veganism benefits

The number of vegans goes up every year, and not only because people are concerned about animal exploitation. There are a number of health reasons to make the switch and cut out meat, dairy, and other animal products:

Improved digestion

Vegan staples like vegetables and fruit are full of fiber, which is essential for a healthy digestive system. On the other hand, animal-based foods, especially dairy, are known to cause chronic gut problems like constipation and inflammation. When you cut those out of your diet and start eating a lot more vegetables, your digestion will improve significantly. If you didn't eat a lot of fiber before, take it slow. When your body isn't used to a high volume of fiber, it can cause issues like diarrhea. Even chewing really thoroughly can help prevent some of the initial symptoms.

Healthier skin

In addition to fiber, fruit and vegetables are packed with water, which will keep you hydrated. That shows on your skin, which can begin glowing and healing from inflammation very soon after you switch to a vegan diet. Plant-based foods are high in other vitamins and nutrients that your skin loves, like vitamin A and Vitamin E. The best foods for skin include beets, avocados, dark leafy greens, oranges, and apples.

More energy

If you struggle with fatigue, a vegan diet can boost your energy. This is most likely because of your healthier digestion system. When it's working harder to digest meat and dairy, it uses up a lot of your energy store, so all you feel like doing is taking a nap. Plant-based foods are much lighter, digest quicker, and contain energy-boosting nutrients like iron, potassium, calcium, and vitamin E and K. Dark leafy greens are very effective at raising your energy levels.

Protection against genetic diseases

Certain diseases are most likely linked to genetics, like type 2 diabetes. However, some studies show that a plant-based diet might help combat your genes and prevent diseases from developing. This is because of various compounds and antioxidants in plants that fight against free radical cells, which cause cell damage, inflammation, and trigger illnesses.

The vegan diet, which cuts out all animal products, has benefits such as improved energy, protection against diseases, healthier skin, and improved digestion.

Protection against cancer

Studies show that vegans have lower cancer rates than meat-eaters or even vegetarians. In 2012, a study funded by the National Cancer Institute found that vegan women had a 34% lower chance of getting cervical, breast, or ovarian cancer. Another study indicated that people who eat meat are at a *higher* risk of colon and prostate cancers. Cutting out meat and dairy while embracing significantly more vegetables, fruit, and other plant-based foods could provide protection from a variety of cancers.

The problems with a vegan diet

Because veganism is so restrictive, it's worth discussing its downsides. The main concern among nutritionists is that the diet has too many nutritional gaps. There are certain nutrients that are more concentrated in animal products than in plant-based ones; some are even *only* present in animal products. The protein in plants is also not as easily-digestible. The solution is to be very aware of your nutritional intake and take supplements, which we will discuss in a later section.

The other weakness with veganism is that despite its emphasis on plants, it's actually relatively easy to become unhealthy. This is because the vegan diet does *not* eliminate processed foods and sugar. A lot of meat substitutes are extremely-processed and packed with artificial ingredients, so you have to be cautious about how you choose food. Just because it lacks animal products, it doesn't mean it's healthy by default.

The vegan diet food list

While restrictive, the list of food you can eat on the vegan diet has a simple qualification: no animal could have been involved. That leaves open the entire world of plants and any manufactured food that doesn't have an animal product on the ingredient list.

What you can eat:
- All grains (bread, pasta, cereal)
- All vegetables
- All fruit
- Nuts/seeds
- Non-dairy cheese substitutes
- Non-dairy yogurt (soy, coconut milk, etc)
- Nut milks (almond, coconut, cashew, pea, etc)
- Meat substitutes (tofu, tempeh, veggie burgers, etc)

What you can't eat:
- All meat (poultry, red meat, pork, etc)
- All seafood (fish, shellfish, etc)
- All dairy (cow's milk, butter, cream, yogurt, cheese, etc)
- Eggs
- Other animal products (gelatin, honey, etc)

II. COMBINING THE KETOGENIC DIET WITH THE VEGAN DIET

Now that you know what the ketogenic and vegan diets are, it's time to talk about combining them. You'll first learn why you should consider doing it at all and what health benefits can result, as well as concerns that nutritionists have with the diet. We'll then dig into a detailed food list of what's allowed and what supplements you should take.

BENEFITS OF A KETOGENIC VEGAN DIET

You know the benefits of the keto and vegan diets, so it makes sense that many would apply to a diet that uses the principles of both. The science behind why can be somewhat different, however, and the diets actually fix each other's problems. For example, when you're a vegan, it's easy to depend on carbs and processed foods. However, when you add the ketogenic element, you have to cut those out. You begin relying on more vegetables, healthy fats, and plant-based proteins instead. With the ketogenic diet, acidic blood can be a problem, especially if you're diabetic. A high consumption of meat and animal products may play a role, so when you switch to veganism, your blood's acidity levels go down.

Here are some other reasons to combine the ketogenic and vegan diets:

Improved energy

Fatigue can be a problem for both the keto and vegan diets on their own. On the regular keto diet, it's common to eat a lot of meat, which takes time and energy to digest. On the vegan diet, you might eat too much bread and other refined carbs. On the keto vegan diet, both of these foods are eliminated, so meals are lighter and packed with fat and fiber. The energy from these ingredients are dispersed over a longer period of time, while any carbs you do eat (from veggies) burn slowly.

Easier weight loss

Both the ketogenic and vegan diets can make weight loss easier. When you combine these diets, you're eliminating a lot of foods that cause weight gain or make weight loss harder, like bread, pasta, sugar, and other refined carbs. Meals full of vegetables are more satisfying, so you're less likely to overeat. The ketogenic vegan diet also encourages eating foods that help with healthy digestion, like fermented ingredients, which keeps your metabolism moving along.

Better sleep

Quality sleep is essential for good health, and what you eat has a significant impact on your sleep hygiene. On a regular vegan diet or diet high in carbs, all those refined carbs cause your blood sugar to go up and down. This can make sleep difficult. However, when your blood levels are more level and stabilized throughout the day, which happens when you adopt a ketogenic vegan diet, it's easier to fall asleep and you're more likely to stay asleep.

WHAT MAKES THE KETOGENIC VEGAN DIET DIFFICULT

The keto and vegan diets are already challenging on their own, and when you combine them, it gets even harder. Here are the three specific reasons why:

It's one of the most restrictive diets you can follow

When you go on the ketogenic vegan diet, you are cutting out all grains, all dairy, and all meat. There are also quite a few vegetables and fruit you can't eat either, because they contain too many carbs. This type of discipline is hard to maintain, so many people will follow the diet for a few months or a year to reset their health, or they will follow an 80-20 rule, which is when they stick to the rules 80% of the time, and eat whatever they want the other 20%. This can affect the benefits of the diet, but it does make life a lot easier.

Getting protein can be tricky

This is an issue many vegans have, but they're able to find protein in vegetables like lentils. However, when on the ketogenic vegan diet, you can't eat lentils. You can't eat meat, obviously either, or any dairy products. Consuming enough high-quality protein doesn't come naturally on this diet, so you have to be very strategic and intentional about adding foods like tofu, tempeh, nuts, seeds, and vegan egg replacements into your diet.

> **The ketogenic vegan diet has a lot of benefits and can improve problems that arise when you're on just one of the diets, but it has drawbacks such as nutritional gaps. It's also very challenging.**

It can cause nutritional gaps

Nutritionists tend to be very wary of restrictive diets. Cutting out entire food groups can lead to nutritional deficiencies, and the ketogenic vegan diet is no different. You should get tested regularly for key vitamins and minerals like B12, zinc, and so on. In a section coming up, we'll get more into these nutrients and what you can do about getting enough of them.

WHAT YOU CAN EAT ON THE VEGAN KETOGENIC DIET

Since this diet is restrictive, the list of foods you can eat is relatively short. However, there's a lot you can do with these ingredients and as the food industry catches up with how people are eating, there will be more and more products that are acceptable. Next to some of the foods, you'll see labels like "fat" and "protein." This just means they are one of the best sources for these essential nutrients:

Vegetables

- Artichoke hearts
- Asparagus
- Beets
- Bell peppers
- Bok choy
- Broccoli
- Cauliflower
- Celery
- Collard greens
- Cucumbers
- Dark leafy greens
- Eggplants
- Endive
- Garlic
- Mushrooms
- No-sugar added pickles
- Onions
- Radishes
- Sauerkraut
- Sea vegetables
- Shallots
- Tomatoes
- Turnips
- Zucchini

Fruit

- Avocados (fat)
- Blackberries
- Canned green jackfruit
- Coconuts
- Cranberries
- Lemons
- Limes
- Raspberries
- Strawberries
- Watermelon

On the ketogenic vegan diet, you cannot eat any grains, meat, dairy, or food high in carbs. This means relying on low-glycemic veggies like dark leafy greens, sea vegetables, cauliflower, mushrooms, and eggplants. You'll also eat berries, as well as high-fat nuts, seeds, oils, and grain-free, sugar-free cooking and baking supplies.

Nuts/seeds

- Almonds (fat/protein)
- Brazil nuts
- Hemp seeds
- Macadamia nuts (fat)
- Pecans (fat)
- Pumpkin seeds (fat/protein)
- Sunflower seeds (fat/protein)

Oils

- Almond butter (fat/protein)
- Almond oil
- Avocado oil
- Cacao butter (fat)
- Coconut butter (fat)
- Coconut oil (fat)
- Extra-virgin olive oil (fat)
- Flaxseed oil
- Hazelnut butter
- Macadamia nut butter

- Pecan butter
- Sunflower seed butter

- Unsweetened peanut butter

Cooking/baking supplies

- Almond flour
- Apple cider vinegar
- Baking powder
- Baking soda
- Cacao powder
- Coconut flour
- Coconut cream
- Coconut milk (full-fat)
- Dairy-free cheese
- Dairy-free unsweetened yogurt (fat)
- Herbs + spices

- High-quality plant-based protein powder (protein)
- Kelp noodles
- No-sugar added organic condiments (hot sauce, mustard, chili sauce, soy sauce, etc)
- No-sugar vanilla extract
- Nutritional yeast (protein)
- Psyllium husk
- Roasted seaweed
- Tempeh (protein)
- Tofu (protein)

SUPPLEMENTS YOU'LL NEED

Since a ketogenic vegan diet is so restrictive, there are a handful of vitamins and minerals that you might not get enough of. Regular testing should be a part of your visits to the doctor, so you can figure out supplements you need. Why not get those nutrients from food? It isn't always possible because certain ones are found only in animal products. Supplements also are much easier; you don't have to readjust your diet and worry about stopping ketosis.

B12

In nature, B12 is only found in animal products. It's also found in fortified grain products. It is essential for a healthy nervous system, so for a ketogenic vegan to get enough, they need to take a supplement since animal products *and* grain are off-limits. To add more to your diet, consider nutritional yeast and fortified soy milk.

Carnosine

Also found only in animal products, this molecule boosts your mood and can aid endurance, which is important for athletic people. The body does produce it naturally, but studies show that many vegans are low, so a supplement is a good idea.

> In addition to meals full of vegetables, plant-based proteins, and healthy fats, you should take supplements to fill in nutritional gaps, such as B12, creatine, D3, and so on. You should also pay special attention to your electrolytes (calcium, sodium, magnesium, and potassium), which can be low during the first weeks of the diet.

Creatine

An acid stored in the muscles and in high volumes in the brain, creatine is a good energy reserve. It's mostly found in pork, salmon, and beef, so ketogenic vegans won't get creatine from those sources. You'll have to take a supplement, especially if you're trying to gain muscle mass.

Choline

When you're eating a lot of fat, your liver works hard to process it. Choline can help, though the best sources (liver and egg yolks) are both not vegan-friendly. Supplements and sunflower lecithin are your options.

DHA/EPA

DHA is important for the body since it comprises a whopping 97% of the brain's omega-3 fats. EPA regulates a healthy blood flow *and* regulates cellular inflammation. Both are omega-3s that you would normally get from fish oil. However, for vegans, you'll take algal oil, which is where fish get their omega-3s in the first place.

D3

Often referred to as simply vitamin D, D3 is fat soluble and allows the body to absorb calcium and phosphorus, which build and strengthen your bones. Studies also suggest it may be important for your immune system, muscle recovery, and brain. The body produces D3 in sunlight, but many people have low levels. When considering a supplement, make sure it's vegan-friendly and using the D3 found in lichen, not animals.

Iron

Iron is essential for your blood as it helps creates new red blood cells and DNA. Without it, you end up with a weak immune system, anemia, and fatigue. You can get non-heme iron from plants, but heme iron is only found in plants. To get heme, which the body absorbs more easily, a supplement is recommended if your level is low. You can also get it from some fortified plant milks. To help with iron absorption, eat foods rich in vitamin C when you take the supplement.

Protein

While you can get enough protein on a plant-based diets, it can be difficult. If you're finding it hard to reach the levels you want, especially if you're very active and wanting to up your protein for the sake of muscle mass, a protein powder is a good supplement. Rice, hemp, and pea proteins are your options on a ketogenic vegan diet. The three have their pros and cons.

Brown rice powder has all the essential amino acids, but is low in lysine, and is often contaminated by heavy metals. Pea protein has a better amount of lysine, so it's common to mix brown rice and pea protein powder together. Hemp protein also has all nine amino acids, as well as omega-3 and magnesium, but it has the least protein of the three powders. When shopping for powders, avoid ones that contain sweeteners, artificial flavors and colors, veggie oils, gluten, fillers, soy protein, and thickeners.

Zinc

This mineral is essential for your immune system, metabolism, and repairing cells. It's difficult to find zinc in plants, and what's available isn't absorbed very easily. Get tested and if your levels are low, consider a supplement and eat more sprouted nuts and seeds. If you really don't want to take another supplement, consider adding clams and/or oysters to your diet. These are considered "non-sentient" creatures. They are full of both zinc and B12, so you could meet your requirements by eating a serving just once a week.

KEEP YOUR ELECTROLYTES REPLENISHED

In addition to watching your intake of B12, carnosine, and so on, you should make sure your diet is supplying you with enough electrolytes. You might have heard the word "electrolytes" thrown around a lot in commercials for sports drinks, but what are they exactly? These are minerals that are essential for a huge variety of bodily functions, including energy production, blood pressure regulation, and immune response. When you're first starting on the ketogenic vegan diet, you lose more water than usual, and as a result, you lose more electrolytes. It's very important to keep these replenished. Here's a list and what foods they can be found in:

Calcium

The body needs this mineral to build strong, healthy bones, as well as perform proper blood clotting and muscle contraction. Deficiency can be hard to spot until it's severe, but watch out for constant fatigue, brittle bones, and trouble building muscle. On a non-vegan diet, you would get calcium from dairy, but on the ketogenic vegan diet, eat lots of dark leafy greens, unsweetened coconut milk, and broccoli.

Sodium

Sodium helps aid nerve and muscle function. It also keeps other electrolytes in proper balance. If you aren't getting enough, you might experience muscle spasms, cramps, dizziness, and fatigue. Thankfully, sodium is an easy electrolyte to replenish; simply use a high-quality salt in your cooking.

Potassium

Potassium balances sodium, so your blood pressure stays at a healthy level, and also regulates fluids and minerals in your cells. If you're feeling tired all the time and experiencing cramping, bloating, and/or constipation, you might be low in potassium. The highest sources are not acceptable on the ketogenic vegan diet, so be sure to get them from dark leafy greens, mushrooms, avocados, and nuts.

Magnesium

This mineral keeps your immune system strong and your nerves and muscles functioning. It's also essential for quality sleep. Deficiency symptoms include fatigue, anxiety, nausea, and loss of appetite. You can get magnesium in dark leafy greens, spinach, almonds, and avocado.

III. EVERYTHING YOU NEED TO KNOW TO SUCCEED ON THE KETOGENIC VEGAN DIET

We've just covered a lot of information about the ketogenic vegan diet. As you can tell, it's not the easiest diet ever, but it has a lot of benefits that are unique. In this section, let's break down everything we learned into a comprehensive guide you can return to again and again when you're feeling confused or worried that you've gone off-track.

REMEMBER THE FIVE ESSENTIALS

When you're starting on the ketogenic vegan diet, it can be tricky to remember everything you're supposed to do. If you weren't on either the keto diet or the vegan diet, it's an especially big transition. When you get overwhelmed, remember there are five main things to focus on. Write them down and hang them on your fridge and cupboards. Once you have these essentials locked down in your brain, you'll be off to a great start:

- #1: No animal products
- #2: No grains
- #3: Eat only 20 grams of net carbs every day
- #4: Eat between 0.4-0.6 grams of protein per pound of your body weight every day
- #5: Get tested for nutrients and take supplements if needed

KNOW WHERE TO GET YOUR FAT, BUT WATCH OUT FOR NUTS AND SEEDS

We could have put "eat lots of fat" into the list of five essentials and brought it up to six, but we believe that you'll definitely remember how important fat is if you're on the ketogenic vegan diet. However, *where* you get your fat is just as important, since many of the normal sources are off-limits. You'll be relying on vegan sources, like avocado, coconut products, olives and olive oil, red palm oil, hemp seeds, and macadamia nuts.

Other nuts and seeds are high in fat, too, but you want to very careful about not overdoing it. It's all too easy to start shoving down handfuls of nuts and seeds when you're trying to eat enough fat, but these are intended only for snacks and as meal-toppings. Why? They contain a lot of calories, first of all, and their carbs add up. They also contain too much omega-6, a fatty acid that can cause an imbalance with omega-3, which over time leads to health problems like raised blood pressure, obesity, and even cancer. To avoid these issues, be sure to get your fat from a variety of sources.

PREPARE FOR THE "KETO FLU"

If you're starting the ketogenic vegan diet from scratch or transitioning from a basic vegan diet, you will most likely experience carb withdrawal. This is affectionately known as the "keto flu," because the symptoms resemble coming down with a flu. For the first week or two, you might feel tired, irritable, and nauseated as your body gets used to missing carbs and begins to rely on the fat you're eating instead. Here are some tips on how to make this process less uncomfortable:

Stay hydrated

As we mentioned earlier, you lose more water than usual when you're starting ketosis. If you don't pay attention, it's very easy to become dehydrated. Be sure to have water with you wherever you go and sip frequently. You don't want to chug full glasses. Plain water will get boring after a while, so switch in other approved beverages like unsweetened coconut water, unsweetened herbal tea, and unsweetened black tea. You can also add citrus slices to your water. For something hot and nutritious, a mug of vegan-friendly vegetable stock with salt is a great way to stay hydrated and get in your sodium.

Exercise (gently)

Depending on how hard the keto flu is hitting you, exercise may seem out of the question. However, doing *something,* even just some light pilates while you're watching TV, will help ease the body into ketosis. This is because exercises like yoga and light cardio rely on fat for fuel instead of glucose, so engaging in these activities forces your body to transition more quickly.

Take some MCT oil

Medium-chain triglycerides encourage ketosis more than long-chain triglycerides, making them perfect for the ketogenic vegan diet. Shortened to MCT, these fats can be found in coconut products. You can even find concentrated MCT oil, but the manufacturing process is often sketchy. It's better to just use a high-quality coconut oil to speed up the process, if you're struggling with the keto flu. Mix just two teaspoons into a glass of water every morning.

Eat some clean carbs

The keto flu is the body going through carb withdrawal and depending on how carb-heavy your diet was before, it might be a real challenge. If you find your symptoms disrupting your life, it's okay to slow down a little and treat your symptoms with some clean carbs. Sweet potatoes, grapes, and nectarines are especially good, because they're full of other great nutrients, too. You don't want to go back to refined carbs. Eating clean carbs will slow down the ketosis process a little, but you will feel much better and more motivated to power through to the end of the keto flu.

The ketogenic vegan diet can seem complicated, so it's important to remember the essentials, such as getting your fat from the best sources, preparing for the keto flu, and keeping a food diary to track your progress and nutrients.

KEEP A FOOD DIARY

Food diaries are very useful when you're watching what you eat, and when you're on a diet where your fat and carb percentages matter so much, writing stuff down is even more important. It can also help you keep track of your progress. Here are some ideas on what to record:

What you ate that day

Every food diary will include what you ate over the course of the day. You can be organized and keep separate sections for breakfast, lunch, dinner, and snacks, or you can just keep a list of everything. It's up to you. App-based food journals will even record the number of calories and macronutrients.

Your ketone levels

When you're starting on the diet, tracking your ketone levels can help you figure out when you hit ketosis. Using one of the methods we discussed earlier (urine strips, breath tests, or blood meters), you can find out your level and write it down. As you enter ketosis and stay there, those levels will go down, because your body is using the ketones. At this point, you might decide to stop tracking.

Your mood

When you stop eating carbs and change your diet significantly, your mood will change, too. If you experience the keto flu, you'll probably be recording your symptoms, but once it starts to improve and the effects of your new diet set in, you'll start seeing a positive change. Write down any changes in your ability to concentrate, irritability, and so on.

How your body feels

Your diet affects your mind and body, so it's a good idea to record how you feel physically. This way, you can figure out if a certain food doesn't agree with you, if you're still hungry and need to eat more during the day, and if you're losing or gaining weight. You should also record your energy levels, since fatigue is a sign that something isn't quite right with your diet.

IT'S NOT ABOUT A NUMBER, IT'S ABOUT HEALTH

Lots of people go on the ketogenic vegan diet because they want to lose weight for one reason or another. However, your health encompasses so much more than just a number on the scale. If you find yourself losing weight, but you're experiencing negative effects like fatigue, weakness, or hunger, something is wrong. Your diet should fuel and strengthen your diet. Learn to listen to what it needs, regardless of what you're hearing about "ideal body weights" from magazines or fitness gurus. You may not achieve your goal weight on this diet, but you might achieve something better: a healthy mind and body.

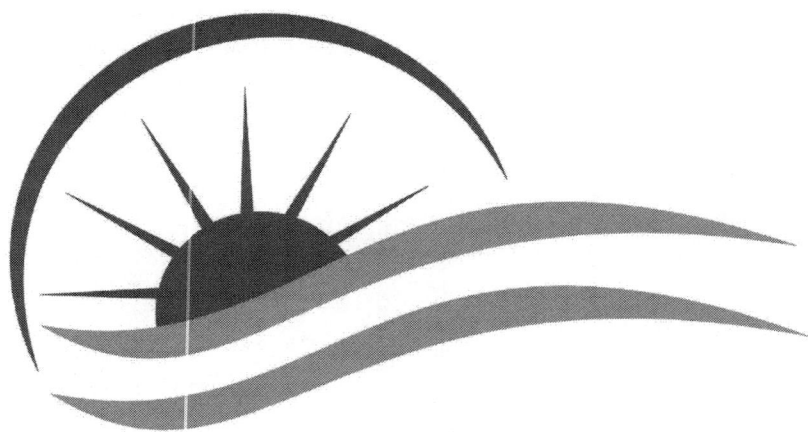

BREAKFAST RECIPES

Contents

Fudge Oats 28

Lemon Pancakes 29

Curried Tofu Scramble 30

Cauliflower and Greens Smoothie Bowl 31

Maple Oatmeal 32

Cinnamon Chocolate Smoothie 33

Flaxseed Waffles 34

Green Coffee Shake 35

Bagels 36

Hemp Heart Porridge 37

Berries Smoothie.. 38

Zucchini Cauliflower Fritters 39

Stuffed Avocado... 40

Sage and Cheddar Waffles 41

Maple Oatmeal Breakfast Bites 42

Coconut Porridge 43

Omelet 44

Doughnuts.. 45

Gingerbread Muffins... 46

Spinach and Tofu Scramble.. 47

Fudge Oats

Serves: 2 / Preparation time: 8 hours and 5 minutes / Cooking time: 0 minutes

½ cup Hemp Hearts

1 tablespoon chia seed

2 tablespoons cacao powder, unsweetened

1/8 teaspoon salt

2 teaspoons erythritol sweetener

½ teaspoon vanilla extract, unsweetened

1 tablespoon almond butter

2/3 cup coconut milk, full-fat and unsweetened

- Place all the ingredients except for milk in a large container, stir until combined and let rest in the refrigerator for 8 hours.
- Then pour in milk and stir well until oats reach to desired consistency.
- Divide evenly among serving bowls and serve.

Per Serving: Net Carbs: 8.5g; Calories: 422; Total Fat: 31g; Saturated Fat: 9.5g; Protein: 18.9g; Carbs: 18g; Fiber: 9.5g; Sugar: 2.2g

Percentage of Calories: Total Fat: 71%; Protein: 15%; Carbs: 14%;

Lemon Pancakes

Serves: 4 / Preparation time: 5 minutes / Cooking time: 30 minutes

1/4 cup coconut flour

1 tablespoon whole Psyllium husks

1/8 teaspoon salt

1 tablespoon erythritol sweetener

1/2 teaspoon baking powder

2 tablespoons coconut butter, melted

1/2 teaspoon vanilla extract, unsweetened

1 tablespoon lemon juice

1 tablespoon coconut oil

5 tablespoons coconut milk, unsweetened

- Place a non-stick skillet pan over medium-low heat, grease with oil and let heat.
- In the meantime, stir together flour, Psyllium husk, salt, and baking powder until mixed.
- Stir the remaining ingredients in another large bowl and then stir in flour mixture, 2 tablespoons at a time, until well incorporated and stiff dough comes together.
- Divide the dough into four portions, then shape into balls and flatten according to the desired thickness of a pancake.
- Transfer a pancake to the heated pan and cook for 5 minutes per side or until nicely golden brown and cooked through.
- Cook remaining pancakes in the same manner and serve straightaway.

Per Serving: Net Carbs: 1.3g; Calories: 108; Total Fat: 10.2g; Saturated Fat: 3g; Protein: 1.5g; Carbs: 2.5g; Fiber: 1.2g; Sugar: 2g

Percentage of Calories: Total Fat: 85%; Protein: 6%; Carbs: 9%;

Curried Tofu Scramble

14-ounce firm tofu, pressed and drained

1 large red pepper, cored diced

6-ounce mushrooms, sliced

1 cup chopped arugula

1 cup chopped spinach

½ of a medium white onion, peeled and diced

3 tablespoons avocado oil

For seasoning:

1/2 teaspoon garlic powder

1/4 teaspoon black salt

1/2 teaspoon curry powder

1/4 teaspoon turmeric

1/4 teaspoon garam masala

1/2 teaspoon cumin

1/4 teaspoon coriander

1/4 teaspoon paprika

1 tablespoon water

- Place a large skillet pan over medium heat, add oil and onion and cook for 5 minutes or until softened.
- Then add mushrooms and peppers and continue cooking for 10 minutes.
- Push cooked vegetables to one side of the pan, add tofu in the other side, then break into small pieces and cook for 3 minutes or more until sauté and hot.
- In the meantime, stir together all the ingredients for seasoning until smooth.
- Pour the seasoning mixture over tofu, toss until evenly coated and then mix with vegetables.
- Add remaining ingredients, stir well and continue cooking for 5 minutes or until greens wilt.
- Serve straightaway.

Per Serving: Net Carbs: 6.8g; Calories: 179; Total Fat: 13g; Saturated Fat: 2g; Protein: 7.2g; Carbs: 8.5g; Fiber: 1.7g; Sugar: 0g

Percentage of Calories: Total Fat: 65%; Protein: 16%; Carbs: 19%;

Cauliflower and Greens Smoothie Bowl

Serves: 2 / Preparation time: 5 minutes / Cooking time: 0 minutes

3 tablespoons hemp hearts and more for garnishing

1 cup blueberries

1/2 cup cauliflower florets, steamed,

1/2 cup diced zucchini

1 cup spinach leaves

1 teaspoon ground cinnamon

1 tablespoon almond butter

2 tablespoons avocado oil

1 cup coconut milk, unsweetened and full-fat

- Place all the ingredients in a blender and blend until smooth.
- Divide smoothie between two bowls, garnish with hemp hearts and serve.

Per Serving: Net Carbs: 10g; Calories: 341; Total Fat: 25g; Saturated Fat: 3g; Protein: 12g; Carbs: 17g; Fiber: 7g; Sugar: 9.5g

Percentage of Calories: Total Fat: 66%; Protein: 14%; Carbs: 20%;

Maple Oatmeal

Serves: 4 / Preparation time: 5 minutes / Cooking time: 30 minutes

4 tablespoons chia seeds

1/4 cup sunflower seeds

1/2 cup walnuts

1/2 cup pecans

1/4 cup coconut flakes

3/8 teaspoon stevia powder

1/2 teaspoon ground cinnamon

1 teaspoon maple flavoring

4 ½ cup almond milk, unsweetened

- Place sunflower seeds, nuts and seeds in a food processor and pulse for 3 to 4 times or until crumbled.
- Tip the mixture in a large pot, add remaining ingredients, stir well and then simmer over low heat for 20 to 30 minutes or until oatmeal thickens to desired level.
- Let oats cool slightly and then serve.

Per Serving: Net Carbs: 3.4g; Calories: 397; Total Fat: 34.5g; Saturated Fat: 4.6g; Protein: 9.25g; Carbs: 12.4g; Fiber: 9g; Sugar: 1.6g

Percentage of Calories: Total Fat: 78%; Protein: 10%; Carbs: 12%;

Cinnamon Chocolate Smoothie

Serves: 1 / Preparation time: 5 minutes / Cooking time: 0 minutes

1/2 of a medium avocado

2 teaspoons cacao powder, unsweetened

1 tablespoon erythritol sweetener

1 teaspoon cinnamon powder

1/4 teaspoon vanilla extract, unsweetened

1 teaspoon avocado oil

3/4 cup coconut milk, full-fat and unsweetened

- Place all the ingredients in a blender and pulse until smooth.
- Serve smoothie straightaway.

Per Serving: Net Carbs: 2.6g; Calories: 159; Total Fat: 13.2g; Saturated Fat: 0g; Protein: 2g; Carbs: 8g; Fiber: 5.4g; Sugar: 0g

Percentage of Calories: Total Fat: 75%; Protein: 5%; Carbs: 20%;

Flaxseed Waffles

Serves: 4 / Preparation time: 10 minutes / Cooking time: 20 minutes

2 cups grounded flaxseed

1 teaspoon sea salt

2 teaspoons ground cinnamon

1 tablespoon baking powder

1/3 cup avocado oil

5 eggs

½ cup water

- Switch on waffle maker and let heat over medium heat setting.
- In the meantime, stir together flax seed, salt, and baking powder until combined, set aside until required.
- Crack eggs in another bowl, add oil and water and blend at high speed until foamy.
- Stir the eggs mixture into flax seed mixture until incorporated and let sit for 5 minutes.
- Then stir in cinnamon, scoop 1/4th of the mixture into waffle maker, shut with lid and cook.
- Prepare remaining waffles in the same manner and serve.

Per Serving: Net Carbs: 2g; Calories: 556.5; Total Fat: 46g; Saturated Fat: 6g; Protein: 18g; Carbs: 16.7g; Fiber: 15g; Sugar: 1.6g

Percentage of Calories: Total Fat: 75%; Protein: 13%; Carbs: 12%;

Green Coffee Shake

Serves: 4 / Preparation time: 5 minutes / Cooking time: 0 minutes

1½ cup brewed coffee, chilled

1 tablespoon green powder, vanilla-flavored

2 tablespoons almond butter

14-ounce coconut milk, full-fat and unsweetened

- Place all the ingredients in a blender and pulse at high speed until smooth.
- Divide smoothie between glasses and serve.

Per Serving: Net Carbs: 2g; Calories: 73.7; Total Fat: 6g; Saturated Fat: 2g; Protein: 1.6g; Carbs: 3.3g; Fiber: 1g; Sugar: 0.5g

Percentage of Calories: Total Fat: 73%; Protein: 9%; Carbs: 18%;

Bagels

Serves: 1 / Preparation time: 5 minutes / Cooking time: 30 minutes

1/2 cup ground flax seed

1 teaspoon salt

1 teaspoon baking powder

1/2 cup tahini

1/4 cup Psyllium husks

1 cup water

Sesame seeds for garnish

- Place pork in a 6-quart slow cooker and switch it on.

Per Serving: Net Carbs: 2.1g; Calories: 212; Total Fat: 16.5g; Saturated Fat: 3g; Protein: 6.4g; Carbs: 9.5g; Fiber: 7.4g; Sugar: 1g

Percentage of Calories: Total Fat: 70%; Protein: 12%; Carbs: 18%;

Hemp Heart Porridge

¼ cup almond flour

2 tablespoons ground flax seed

1 tablespoon chia seeds

½ cup Hemp Hearts and more for topping

1 tablespoon swerve sweetener

½ teaspoon ground cinnamon

¾ teaspoon vanilla extract, unsweetened

1 cup almond milk, unsweetened

- Place all the ingredients except for almonds in a small saucepan and stir until combined.
- Place the pan over medium heat and bring the mixture to a light boil.
- Boil for 2 minutes, then remove the pan from heat and stir in almond flour until well mixed.
- Garnish with hemp hearts and serve.

Per Serving: Net Carbs: 5.6g; Calories: 504; Total Fat: 40g; Saturated Fat: 3.7g; Protein: 24g; Carbs: 12.6g; Fiber: 7g; Sugar: 1.8g

Percentage of Calories: Total Fat: 71%; Protein: 19%; Carbs: 10%;

Berries Smoothie

Serves: 2 / Preparation time: 5 minutes / Cooking time: 30 minutes

1 cup baby spinach

3 cups frozen strawberries

3 cups frozen blackberries

1 tablespoon avocado oil

2 ½ cups coconut milk, full-fat and unsweetened

- Place all the ingredients in a blender and pulse until smooth.
- Divide smoothie between two glasses and serve.

Per Serving: Net Carbs: 6.3g; Calories: 167.5; Total Fat: 13.4g; Saturated Fat: 6.8g; Protein: 2g; Carbs: 9.6g; Fiber: 3.3g; Sugar: 5g

Percentage of Calories: Total Fat: 62%; Protein: 34%; Carbs: 4%;

Zucchini Cauliflower Fritters

Serves: 4 / Preparation time: 10 minutes / Cooking time: 25 minutes

1/4 cup almond flour

3 cups grated cauliflower

2 medium zucchini

½ teaspoon sea salt

¼ teaspoon ground black pepper

2 tablespoons coconut oil

- Place zucchini in a microwave proof bowl, cover with plastic wrap and microwave for 3 to 5 minutes or until steamed.
- Wrap zucchini into a cheese cloth and twist the cloth tightly to squeeze moisture as much as possible.
- Squeeze cauliflower in the same manner and then transfer vegetables to a bowl.
- Add remaining ingredients except for oil, stir until well mixed and then shape the mixture into 8 patties.
- Place a skillet pan over medium heat, grease with oil and when hot, add patties in a single layer.
- Cook for 2 to 3 minutes per side or until patties are nicely brown.
- Cook remaining patties in the same manner and serve.

Per Serving: Net Carbs: 4.2g; Calories: 137.5; Total Fat: 10.5g; Saturated Fat: 6g; Protein: 3g; Carbs: 7.5g; Fiber: 3.3g; Sugar: 4.3g

Percentage of Calories: Total Fat: 69%; Protein: 9%; Carbs: 22%;

Stuffed Avocado

Serves: 4 / Preparation time: 10 minutes / Cooking time: 5 minutes

2 large avocados, pitted and halved

1/2 cup cauliflower rice

1 chipotle chili in adobo sauce, minced

1/2 cup crushed walnuts

1/2 teaspoon sea salt

1/2 teaspoon cumin

2 tablespoons avocado oil

1 tablespoon adobo sauce

1 cup tomato salsa, low-carb

2 tablespoons vegan mayonnaise

- Whisk together mayonnaise and adobo sauce until combined and set aside until required.
- Place a medium skillet pan over medium heat, add oil and when hot, add cauliflower and walnuts and stir in salt, chipotle pepper and cumin.
- Cook for 5 minutes or until cauliflower is softened and then spoon the mixture into the avocado.
- Top with salsa and mayonnaise and serve.

Per Serving: Net Carbs: 5.3g; Calories: 336; Total Fat: 31.6g; Saturated Fat: 4g; Protein: 5g; Carbs: 13.9g; Fiber: 8.6g; Sugar: 2g

Percentage of Calories: Total Fat: 88%; Protein: 6%; Carbs: 6%;

Sage and Cheddar Waffles

Serves: 12 / Preparation time: 5 minutes / Cooking time: 45 minutes

1 1/3 cup coconut flour

1/4 teaspoon garlic powder

1/2 teaspoon salt

3 teaspoons baking powder

4 tablespoons arrowroot power

1 teaspoon sage

4 tablespoons avocado oil

2 cups coconut milk, unsweetened

1/2 cup water

1 cup shredded vegan cheddar cheese

- Switch on the waffle iron, grease with oil and let preheat over medium heat.
- In the meantime, stir together flour, garlic powder, salt, baking powder, arrowroot powder, and sage until mixed.
- Whisk together avocado oil, milk and water until smooth and then stir in flour mixture, 2 tablespoons at a time, until well incorporated.
- Fold in cheese, then scoop 1/3 cup of the batter in a waffle iron, shut with lid and cook.
- Cook remaining waffles in the same manner and serve.

Per Serving: Net Carbs: 4.8g; Calories: 165.5; Total Fat: 14g; Saturated Fat: 3.4g; Protein: 4.5g; Carbs: 5.4g; Fiber: 1.5g; Sugar: 0.6g

Percentage of Calories: Total Fat: 76%; Protein: 10.8%; Carbs: 13%;

Maple Oatmeal Breakfast Bites

Serves: 10 / Preparation time: 10 minutes / Cooking time: 0 minutes

1/4 cup hulled hemp hearts

2 tablespoons chia seeds

3 tablespoons erythritol sweetener

1/4 cup protein powder

1 tablespoon avocado oil

1/4 cup peanut butter, unsweetened

- Place all the ingredients in a bowl and stir until incorporated.
- Shape dough into 10 balls, each of 1 tablespoon size.
- Let balls chill in refrigerator for 30 minutes and then serve.

Per Serving: Net Carbs: 1.7g; Calories: 117.5; Total Fat: 8g; Saturated Fat: 1.24g; Protein: 7g; Carbs: 3.2g; Fiber: 1.5g; Sugar: 1.1g

Percentage of Calories: Total Fat: 64%; Protein: 25%; Carbs: 11%;

Coconut Porridge

Serves: 6 / Preparation time: 5 minutes / Cooking time: 15 minutes

1/4 cup coconut flour

1 cup shredded coconut, full-fat and unsweetened

1/2 teaspoon cinnamon

1/4 teaspoon nutmeg

1/4 cup Psyllium husks

30 drops stevia liquid

1 teaspoon vanilla extract, unsweetened

20 drops monk fruit liquid

2 cups coconut milk, unsweetened

2 2/3 cups water

- Switch on instant pot, press sauté button, and then wait until hot and add coconut into the inner pot.
- Cook coconut for 5 minutes or until toasted, then pour in milk and water and stir well.
- Press the cancel button, shut instant pot with lid, then press pressure button to set at high pressure and cook for 0 minutes.
- When the instant pot beeps, release pressure naturally, then open instant pot and stir well.
- Serve straightaway.

Per Serving: Net Carbs: 2g; Calories: 305; Total Fat: 25g; Saturated Fat: 23g; Protein: 3g; Carbs: 17g; Fiber: 11g; Sugar: 1g

Percentage of Calories: Total Fat: 74%; Protein: 4%; Carbs: 22%;

Omelet

Serves: 1 / Preparation time: 5 minutes / Cooking time: 15 minutes

1/4 cup lupini flour

1/8 teaspoon dehydrated onion

1/4 teaspoon garlic powder

¼ teaspoon baking powder

1/8 teaspoon black salt

1/8 teaspoon ground black pepper

1 tablespoon nutritional yeast

1 tablespoon avocado oil

- Place a medium skillet pan over medium-low heat, add oil and let preheat.
- In the meantime, stir together remaining ingredients until smooth and then pour into the center of the heated pan.
- Spread the batter into 6 to 7-inch diameter pancake, then cover the pan and cook for 5 to 10 minutes or until cooked through from center.
- Then carefully flip the omelet, remove the pan from heat and let omelet sit in the pan for 2 minutes.
- Slide omelet to the serving plate and serve.

Per Serving: Net Carbs: 3g; Calories: 302; Total Fat: 20.5g; Saturated Fat: 1.9g; Protein: 14.3g; Carbs: 15.1g; Fiber: 12.1g; Sugar: 1g

Percentage of Calories: Total Fat: 61%; Protein: 19%; Carbs: 20%;

Doughnuts

Serves: 6 / Preparation time: 10 minutes / Cooking time: 40 minutes

3 tablespoon coconut flour

1/8 teaspoon salt

1/4 teaspoon ground cinnamon

1/8 teaspoon nutmeg

1/4 teaspoon baking powder

3 tablespoons erythritol sweetener

1 tablespoon Psyllium Husk

1 teaspoon vanilla extract, extract

1 tablespoon apple cider vinegar

1/2 cup coconut manna

1/2 cup and 2 tablespoons almond milk, unsweetened

- Set oven to 350 degrees F and let preheat.
- In the meantime, grease six dough pans and set aside until required.
- Prepare a double boiler by bringing a medium saucepan filled with water to bowl, place a heatproof bowl in it.
- Then whisk in vanilla, vinegar, coconut manna, and milk until smooth and let heat for 5 minutes.
- Remove the bowl from double boiler, then stir in remaining ingredients until smooth and let the mixture sit for 5 minutes.
- Evenly divide the mixture among dough pans, smooth the top and bake into the heated oven for 20 to 30 minutes or until edges are nicely brown and inserted toothpick into the doughnuts come out clean.
- When done, take out dough from the pan and let cool completely before serving.

Per Serving: Net Carbs: 2.1g; Calories: 152.3; Total Fat: 12.7g; Saturated Fat: 4g; Protein: 2g; Carbs: 7.5g; Fiber: 5.4g; Sugar: 3g

Percentage of Calories: Total Fat: 62%; Protein: 34%; Carbs: 4%;

Gingerbread Muffins

Serves: 8 / Preparation time: 10 minutes / Cooking time: 35 minutes

1/2 cup coconut flour

1/2 cup ground flax seeds

1 1/2 teaspoon grated ginger

1/4 cup swerve sweetener

1 1/2 teaspoon ground cinnamon

1/4 teaspoon ground nutmeg

1/4 teaspoon ground cloves

1/4 teaspoon ground allspice

1 teaspoon vanilla extract, unsweetened

2 tablespoons avocado oil

3/4 cup almond milk, unsweetened

- Set oven to 375 degrees F and let preheat.
- In the meantime, line a 5 silicon muffin pans with paper liners and set aside until required.
- In a bowl, whisk together all the ingredients, except for cinnamon, nutmeg, cloves, and allspice, until smooth.
- Stir together remaining ingredients, then add to flour mixture and scoop into prepared muffin cups.
- Place muffin cups into the oven and bake for 30 to 35 minutes or until top is nicely golden brown and inserted wooden skewer into each muffin comes out clean.
- When done, cool muffins on wire rack completely, then run a knife along the edges and take out muffins to serve.

Per Serving: Net Carbs: 2.4g; Calories: 167; Total Fat: 12.8g; Saturated Fat: 5g; Protein: 3.8g; Carbs: 10.9g; Fiber: 8.5g; Sugar: 2g

Percentage of Calories: Total Fat: 66%; Protein: 9%; Carbs: 25%;

Spinach and Tofu Scramble

Serves: 8 / Preparation time: 5 minutes / Cooking time: 20 minutes

14-ounce firm tofu, pressed

1 cup baby spinach

3 grape tomatoes

2 tablespoons diced yellow onion

1/2 teaspoon garlic powder

1/2 teaspoons salt

1/2 teaspoon turmeric

1 1/2 tablespoons nutritional yeast

3 tablespoons avocado oil

3 ounces vegan cheddar cheese

- Place a skillet pan over medium heat, add 1 tablespoon oil and when oil, add onion and cook for 5 minutes or until softened.
- Then add tofu, crumble with a potato masher, then drizzle with remaining oil and season with garlic powder, salt, and turmeric.
- Stir well until coated and cook for 5 to 8 minutes or until most of the cooking liquid is evaporated.
- Add spinach, tomato, onion, and cheese and cook for 3 minutes or more until spinach leaves wilts and cheese is melted.
- Serve straightaway.

Per Serving: Net Carbs: 4.7g; Calories: 224.7; Total Fat: 17.5g; Saturated Fat: 5.5g; Protein: 10g; Carbs: 6.8g; Fiber: 2.1g; Sugar: 2g

Percentage of Calories: Total Fat: 70%; Protein: 18%; Carbs: 12%;

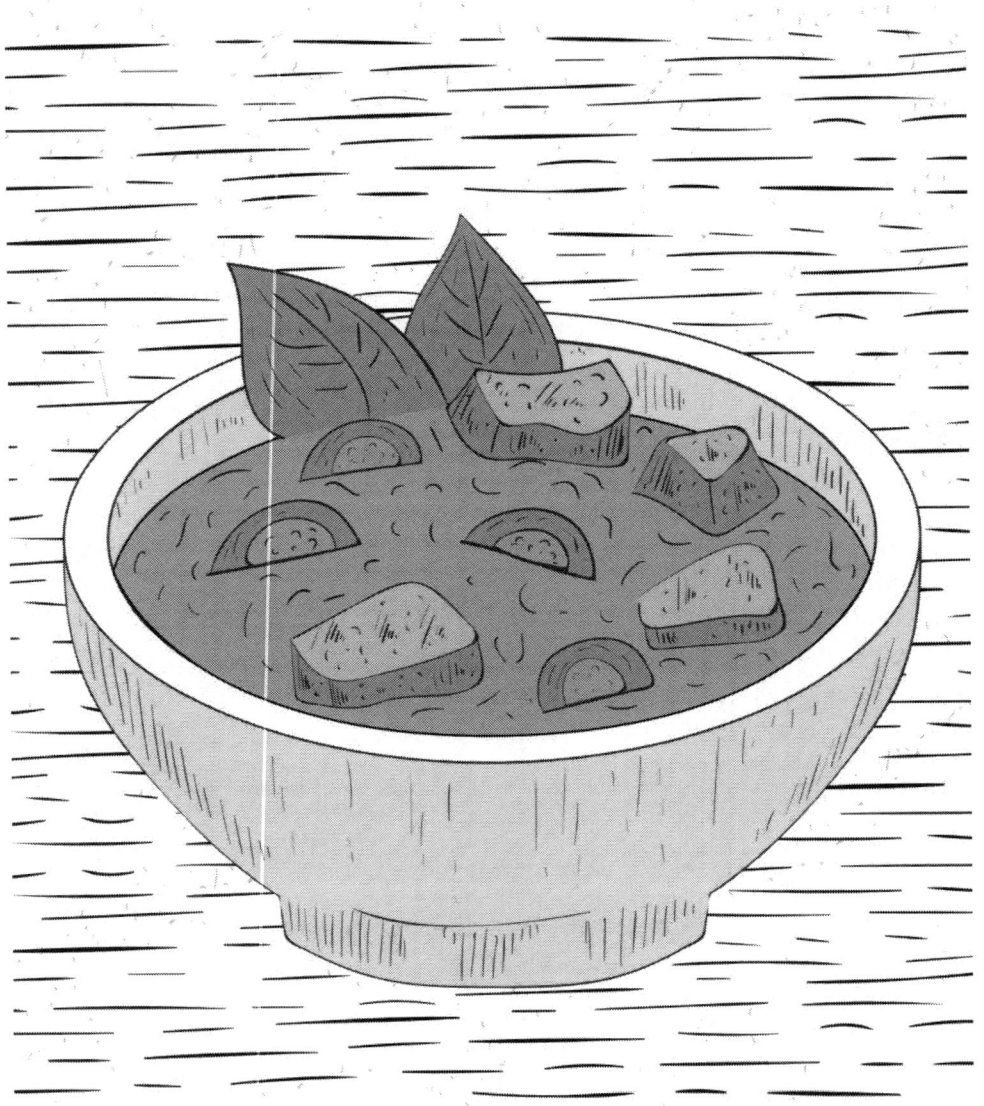

SOUPS AND SALADS RECIPES

Contents

Thai Soup 50

Red Curry Cauliflower Soup 51

Cream of Mushroom Soup 52

Roasted Red Pepper Soup 53

Superfood Keto 54

Green Soup 55

Avocado Arugula Salad 56

Triple Green Kale Salad 57

Tomato Mushroom Spaghetti Squash 58

Ginger Coleslaw 59

Caesar Salad 60

Curry Noodle Bowls 61

Zucchini Salad 62

Crack Slaw 63

Halloumi Salad 64

Egg Roll Bowl 65

Cucumber Salad 66

Spinach and Artichoke Soup 67

Creamy Broccoli Soup 68

Kale and Spinach Soup 69

Thai Soup

Serves: 6 / Preparation time: 5 minutes / Cooking time: 20 minutes

16 ounces tofu, drained and pressed

½ cup shiitake mushrooms, sliced

1/2 of medium red onion, sliced

1 ½ teaspoon minced garlic

2 tablespoon red chili paste

4 tablespoons avocado oil

1 1/2 cups vegetable broth

12-ounce coconut milk, full-fat and unsweetened

1 lime, juiced

- Place a large saucepan over medium heat, add oil, mushroom, onion, and garlic and cook for 3 to 5 minutes or until lightly cooked.
- Then reduce heat to medium-low, add tofu, red chili paste, and lime juice and pour in vegetable broth and coconut milk.
- Stir until mixed and simmer soup for 15 minutes or until done.
- Serve straightaway.

Per Serving: Net Carbs: 5.3g; Calories: 162.2; Total Fat: 12.8g; Saturated Fat: 2.3g; Protein: 6g; Carbs: 5.6g; Fiber: 0.3g; Sugar: 3.3g

Percentage of Calories: Total Fat: 71%; Protein: 15%; Carbs: 14%;

Red Curry Cauliflower Soup

Serves: 6 / Preparation time: 10 minutes / Cooking time: 35 minutes

1 large head of cauliflower, cut into florets

1 medium white onion, peeled and diced

½ teaspoon ground black pepper

4 tablespoons Thai red curry paste

1 tablespoon lemon zest

1 ½ teaspoon sea salt

6 tablespoons avocado oil

4 cups vegetable broth

14-ounces coconut milk, unsweetened and full-fat

Hot sauce for serving

- Set oven to 400 degrees F and let preheat.
- In the meantime, spread cauliflower and onion on a large baking tray, lined with parchment paper, then season with salt and black pepper and drizzle with 3 tablespoons oil.
- Toss until combined, then place the baking tray into the oven and bake for 20 minutes or until done.
- When done, let cauliflower and onion cool, then transfer to a blender and add remaining ingredients, except for coconut milk.
- Pulse until smooth, then transfer soup into a medium saucepan and stir in coconut milk.
- Place saucepan over medium heat, bring the soup to simmer, then reduce heat to low and cook for 10 to 15 minutes.
- Ladle soup into serving bowls, drizzle with hot sauce and serve.

Per Serving: Net Carbs: 8.5g; Calories: 193.6; Total Fat: 15g; Saturated Fat: 3g; Protein: 2.4g; Carbs: 12g; Fiber: 3.5g; Sugar: 5.5g

Percentage of Calories: Total Fat: 70%; Protein: 5%; Carbs: 25%;

Cream of Mushroom Soup

Serves: 6 / Preparation time: 5 minutes / Cooking time: 60 minutes

5 cups chopped mushrooms

½ cup chopped white onion

½ teaspoon minced garlic

½ teaspoon salt

14 teaspoon dried thyme

¼ cup avocado oil

½ teaspoon ground black pepper

32-ounce vegetable broth

2 cups coconut milk, unsweetened and full-fat

4-ounce tofu, pressed and crumbled

- Place a large saucepan over medium heat, add oil and when hot, add mushroom, onion, and garlic and cook for 10 minutes or until vegetables are tender.
- Stir in salt, black pepper, and thyme and continue cooking for 1 minute or until fragrant.
- Add remaining ingredients, stir until mixed, then reduce heat to a low level and cook for 45 minutes or until cooked through, stirring constantly.
- When done, ladle soup into bowls and serve.

Per Serving: Net Carbs: 6.8g; Calories: 453; Total Fat: 44.2g; Saturated Fat: 27.3g; Protein: 5.9g; Carbs: 7.7g; Fiber: 0.9g; Sugar: 2.5g

Percentage of Calories: Total Fat: 88%; Protein: 5%; Carbs: 7%;

Roasted Red Pepper Soup

Serves: 6 / Preparation time: 5 minutes / Cooking time: 25 minutes

5 cups cauliflower florets

1/2 cup roasted red pepper, chopped

½ cup chopped shallot

1 teaspoon celery sea salt

1 tablespoon seasoned salt

1 teaspoon paprika

1 pinch crushed red pepper flakes

1/8 teaspoon fresh thyme

1 teaspoon apple cider vinegar

10 tablespoons avocado oil, divided

4 cups vegetable broth

1 cup coconut milk, unsweetened and full-fat

- Place a large saucepan over medium heat, add 4 tablespoons oil and when hot, add shallots and cook for 3 minutes or until softened.
- Add red peppers, sea salt, seasoned salt, paprika, red pepper flakes, and thyme, stir well and cook for 3 minutes.
- Add cauliflower, vinegar, and stock and simmer for 10 to 15 minutes or until cauliflower is soft.
- When done, puree soup using a stick blender until smooth.
- Return pan over medium heat, stir in milk and let cook for 2 minutes or until hot.
- Ladle soup between 6 serving bowls, drizzle with 1 tablespoon oil and serve straight away.

Per Serving: Net Carbs: 11.5g; Calories: 277; Total Fat: 23.1g; Saturated Fat: 3.3g; Protein: 2.7g; Carbs: 14.5g; Fiber: 3g; Sugar: 8.1g

Percentage of Calories: Total Fat: 75%; Protein: 4%; Carbs: 21%;

Superfood Keto

Serves: 6 / Preparation time: 5 minutes / Cooking time: 15 minutes

1 medium head of cauliflower

5.3-ounce watercress

8-ounce frozen spinach

1 medium white onion, peeled and diced

1 teaspoon minced garlic

½ teaspoon ground black pepper

1 bay leaf, crumbled

1 teaspoon salt

4 cups vegetable stock

1 cup coconut milk, unsweetened and full-fat

1/4 cup avocado oil

- Place a large saucepan over medium-high heat, add oil and then add onion and garlic.
- Cook for 3 to 5 minutes or until slightly brown, then add cauliflower and bay leaf and cook for 5 minutes.
- Add spinach and watercress, continue cooking for 3 minutes, then pour in vegetable stock and bring the mixture to boil.
- Pour in coconut milk, season with salt and black pepper and remove the pan from heat.
- Puree soup using an immersion blender until smooth and creamy.
- Let cool the soup slightly, then ladle into bowls and serve.

Per Serving: Net Carbs: 6.8g; Calories: 396.8; Total Fat: 37.6g; Saturated Fat: 3g; Protein: 4.9g; Carbs: 9.7g; Fiber: 2.9g; Sugar: 1.5g

Percentage of Calories: Total Fat: 85%; Protein: 5%; Carbs: 10%;

Green Soup

Serves: 6 / Preparation time: 10 minutes / Cooking time: 30 minutes

6-ounce baby spinach

8-ounce kale

1 1/2 cups chopped broccoli

1 cup chopped cauliflower

1 large white onion, diced

1 ½ teaspoon minced garlic

¾ teaspoon ground black pepper

1/4 cup almond meal

1/4 teaspoon ground cinnamon

1 ½ teaspoon sea salt

1 tablespoon lemon juice

3 tablespoons avocado oil

2 tablespoons coconut cream and more for drizzling

5 cups vegetable stock

¾ cup grated vegan parmesan cheese

- Place a large saucepan over medium heat, add oil and when hot, add onion and garlic and cook on lower heat for 5 minutes or more until softened.
- Then add kale, broccoli, and cauliflower, season with cinnamon and stir to coat.
- Pour in the stock, switch heat to medium level and simmer soup for 25 minutes or until vegetables are softened, covering the pan.
- When the last 5 minutes of cooking time is left, add spinach to soup and cook.
- When done, remove the pan from heat and let soup cool slightly.
- Then stir in remaining ingredients except for cheese and puree soup using an immersion blender.
- Ladle soup into bowl, top with coconut cream and cheese and serve.

Per Serving: Net Carbs: 9.5g; Calories: 597; Total Fat: 50g; Saturated Fat: 18.5g; Protein: 21.4g; Carbs: 15.5g; Fiber: 6g; Sugar: 4g

Percentage of Calories: Total Fat: 75%; Protein: 14%; Carbs: 11%;

Avocado Arugula Salad

Serves: 4 / Preparation time: 5 minutes / Cooking time: 0 minutes

1 ½ pint red cherry tomatoes, halved

5-ounce baby arugula, chopped

2 large avocados, peeled, pitted and diced

1/4 cup diced red onion

6 large basil leaves, sliced

For Vinaigrette:

½ teaspoon minced garlic

1/4 teaspoon ground black pepper

1 tablespoon stevia

1/2 teaspoon Italian seasonings

1/4 teaspoon sea salt

2 tablespoons balsamic vinegar

3 tablespoons avocado oil

1 lemon, juiced

- Place all the ingredients of vinaigrette in a small bowl and whisk until combined.
- Then place salad ingredients in a large bowl, drizzle with prepared vinaigrette and toss until combined.
- Serve straightaway.

Per Serving: Net Carbs: 4.9g; Calories: 229; Total Fat: 68g; Saturated Fat: 2.3g; Protein: 5.7g; Carbs: 13.2g; Fiber: 8.3g; Sugar: 5.2g

Percentage of Calories: Total Fat: 68%; Protein: 10%; Carbs: 23%;

Triple Green Kale Salad

Serves: 4 / Preparation time: 5 minutes / Cooking time: 0 minutes

1 medium avocado, sliced

10-ounce kale, sliced

¼ cup chopped Snow peas

1 teaspoon minced garlic

1 teaspoon grated ginger

½ teaspoon sea salt

2 teaspoons coconut aminos

2 teaspoons apple balsamic vinegar

2 teaspoons sesame oil

4 teaspoons avocado oil

- Place kale leaves in a large bowl, add garlic, ginger, salt, sesame oil, and avocado oil, toss until well coated and then massage gently for few seconds.
- Then add remaining ingredients and toss until just mixed.
- Serve straightaway.

Per Serving: Net Carbs: 7g; Calories: 196; Total Fat: 16g; Saturated Fat: 1g; Protein: 3g; Carbs: 10g; Fiber: 3g; Sugar: 1g

Percentage of Calories: Total Fat: 73%; Protein: 6%; Carbs: 21%;

Tomato Mushroom Spaghetti Squash

Serves: 4 / Preparation time: 5 minutes / Cooking time: 10 minutes

2 spaghetti squash, cooked

1 ½ cups diced tomatoes

8 ounces mushrooms, sliced

2 tablespoons basil leaves

2 teaspoons minced garlic

½ teaspoon ground black pepper

1/8 teaspoon red pepper flakes

1 teaspoon salt

1/4 cup toasted pine nuts

4 tablespoons avocado oil

- Cut each cooked spaghetti squash into the half, then remove seeds and run fork in its flesh, lengthwise, to shred squash, set aside until required.
- Place a large skillet pan over medium heat, add oil and when hot, add mushrooms and cook for 3 to 4 minutes or until softened.
- Then add garlic and cook for 2 minutes or until fragrant, add tomatoes and shredded spaghetti squash, toss well and cook until hot.
- Add remaining ingredients and serve.

Per Serving: Net Carbs: 10.6g; Calories: 243.6; Total Fat: 18.9g; Saturated Fat: 2.5g; Protein: 3g; Carbs: 15.2g; Fiber: 4.6g; Sugar: 8g

Percentage of Calories: Total Fat: 62%; Protein: 34%; Carbs: 4%;

Ginger Coleslaw

Serves: 4 / Preparation time: 1 hour and 5 minutes / Cooking time: 0 minutes

For Coleslaw:

6 cups sliced green cabbage

6 cups sliced red cabbage

1 cup chopped cilantro

3/4 cup green onions, sliced

For Dressing:

1 teaspoon grated ginger

½ teaspoon minced garlic

1 teaspoon ground black pepper

1/4 teaspoon cayenne pepper

10 drops stevia sweetener

2 teaspoons sea salt

2 tablespoons avocado oil

1 teaspoon sesame oil

2 tablespoons apple cider vinegar

2 tablespoons tamari

3 tablespoons lime juice

2 tablespoon almond butter

- Place all the ingredients for dressing in a blender and pulse at high speed until smooth.
- Place coleslaw ingredients in a large bowl, drizzle with dressing and toss until combined.
- Place coleslaw bowl in refrigerator to chill for 1 hour and then serve.

Per Serving: Net Carbs: 9.4g; Calories: 267; Total Fat: 20.2g; Saturated Fat: 2.2g; Protein: 4.7g; Carbs: 16.7g; Fiber: 7.3g; Sugar: 10.5g

Percentage of Calories: Total Fat: 68%; Protein: 7%; Carbs: 25%;

Caesar Salad

Serves: 4 / Preparation time: 10 minutes / Cooking time: 0 minutes

¼ cup hemp seeds

12 cups chopped romaine lettuce

¾ teaspoon sea salt

1 medium avocado, peeled and sliced

1 tablespoon capers

1 ½ teaspoon minced garlic

½ teaspoon ground black pepper

2 teaspoons mustard

3 tablespoons lemon juice

3 tablespoons avocado oil

2 tablespoons water

- Place avocado into a blender, add capers, garlic, salt, black pepper, mustard, lemon juice, oil, and water.
- Tip the dressing in a small bowl, add hemp seeds and stir until mixed.
- Place lettuce in a large bowl, top with prepared dressing and toss until coated.
- Serve straightaway.

Per Serving: Net Carbs: 1.4g; Calories: 223.75; Total Fat: 18.8g; Saturated Fat: 2.6g; Protein: 4g; Carbs: 9.5g; Fiber: 8.1g; Sugar: 2g

Percentage of Calories: Total Fat: 76%; Protein: 7%; Carbs: 17%;

Curry Noodle Bowls

Serves: 2 / Preparation time: 10 minutes / Cooking time: 0 minutes

For Noodles:

0.5ounce pack of Kanten Noodles

1 carrot, peeled and julienned

½ head of medium cauliflower, cut into florets

1 medium red bell pepper, cored and diced

¼ cup chopped cilantro

½ cup mixed greens

For Creamy Curry Sauce:

¼ teaspoon ground ginger

½ teaspoon ground black pepper

2 teaspoons curry powder

1 teaspoon ground turmeric

1½ teaspoons ground coriander

1 teaspoon sea salt

1 teaspoon ground cumin

2 tablespoons apple cider vinegar

¼ cup avocado oil mayonnaise

4 tablespoons avocado oil

¼ cup water

- Boil a couple of cups of water, then pour into a bowl, add noodles and let rest for 5 minutes.
- Then drain noodles and place into a bowl along with carrot, cauliflower, and pepper.
- Place curry sauce ingredients in a blender and pulse until smooth.
- Drizzle the sauce over noodles and vegetables and then toss until well coated.
- Divide green evenly between two plate, top with noodles and serve.

Per Serving: Net Carbs: 8g; Calories: 347.5; Total Fat: 75g; Saturated Fat: 3.6g; Protein: 3.4g; Carbs: 18.2g; Fiber: 6.2g; Sugar: 8.3g

Percentage of Calories: Total Fat: 75%; Protein: 4%; Carbs: 21%;

Zucchini Salad

Serves: 10 / Preparation time: 2 hours and 10 minutes / Cooking time: 0 minutes

1 cup sunflower seeds, shelled

1 cup sliced almonds

1 medium zucchini, thinly spiralized

1 pound shredded cabbage

1 teaspoon stevia drops

3/4 cup avocado oil

1/3 cup apple cider vinegar

- Place cabbage in a large bowl, add almonds and sunflower seeds and toss until mixed.
- Cut zucchini into smaller pieces, add to cabbage and toss until mixed.
- Whisk together stevia, oil, and vinegar in another bowl until combined, then pour the dressing over salad and toss until well mixed.
- Place salad in refrigerator for 2 hours or more until chilled and then serve.

Per Serving: Net Carbs: 2.6g; Calories: 120; Total Fat: 9.3g; Saturated Fat: 1g; Protein: 4g; Carbs: 7.3g; Fiber: 4.7g; Sugar: 2.4g

Percentage of Calories: Total Fat: 65%; Protein: 12%; Carbs: 23%;

Crack Slaw

Serves: 2 / Preparation time: 5 minutes / Cooking time: 10 minutes

4 cups shredded green cabbage

½ teaspoon sesame seeds

1/2 cup macadamia nuts, chopped

1 teaspoon minced garlic

1 teaspoon red chili paste

1 teaspoon apple cider vinegar

2 tablespoons tamari

1 tablespoon sesame oil

1 tablespoon avocado oil

- Whisk together red chili paste, vinegar, tamari, sesame oil and avocado oil in a small bowl and pour into a skillet pan.
- Place skillet pan over medium-low heat, add cabbage and garlic and toss until mixed.
- Cover the pan and cook for 5 minutes or until cabbage starts to tender.
- Then stir until well combined, add nuts and continue cooking for 5 minutes or more until nuts absorb some of the cooking liquid.
- Garnish with sesame seed and serve.

Per Serving: Net Carbs: 7.3g; Calories: 389.7; Total Fat: 34.5g; Saturated Fat: 15.7g; Protein: 5.5g; Carbs: 14.3g; Fiber: 7g; Sugar: 5g

Percentage of Calories: Total Fat: 80%; Protein: 6%; Carbs: 14%;

Halloumi Salad

Serves: 8 / Preparation time: 5 minutes / Cooking time: 10 minutes

1 tablespoon chopped walnuts

1 medium cucumber

5 grape tomatoes

¼ cup baby arugula

½ teaspoon salt

1 tablespoon apple cider vinegar

1 ½ tablespoon avocado oil

3-ounce vegan halloumi cheese

- Cut cheese into 1/3 inch slices.
- Place a griddle pan over medium heat, grease with oil and when hot, grill cheese for 3 to 5 minutes per side.
- Place nuts, cucumber, tomato and arugula in a bowl, top with grilled cheese and season with salt and drizzle with vinegar and oil.
- Serve straightaway.

Per Serving: Net Carbs: 4g; Calories: 233; Total Fat: 47g; Saturated Fat: 24g; Protein: 21g; Carbs: 7g; Fiber: 3g; Sugar: 2g

Percentage of Calories: Total Fat: 80%; Protein: 15%; Carbs: 5%;

Egg Roll Bowl

Serves: 2 / Preparation time: 5 minutes / Cooking time: 25 minutes

4 cups shredded green cabbage

1 cup shredded carrot

2 celery stalks, chopped

1 cup sliced mushrooms

1/2 of medium red onion, peeled and sliced

¼ teaspoon ground black pepper

2 tablespoons tamari

1/4 teaspoon sea salt

4 tablespoons avocado oil

1 teaspoon sesame oil

1 teaspoon sesame seeds

- Place a large skillet pan over medium-high heat, add 2 tablespoons oil and when hot, add onion, carrot, and celery and cook for 5 minutes or until tender.
- Then add cabbage and mushroom, season with salt, black pepper and tamari, drizzle with remaining oil and cook for 10 to 15 minutes or until vegetables are tender-crisp, covering the pan.
- Drizzle with sesame oil and remove the pan from heat.
- Garnish with sesame seeds and serve.

Per Serving: Net Carbs: 11.1g; Calories: 363; Total Fat: 30.2g; Saturated Fat: 3.7g; Protein: 4.5g; Carbs: 18.2g; Fiber: 7.1g; Sugar: 10.7g

Percentage of Calories: Total Fat: 75%; Protein: 5%; Carbs: 20%;

Cucumber Salad

Serves: 4 / Preparation time: 10 minutes / Cooking time: 0 minutes

For The Salad:

2 cups chopped kale

2 cups chopped spinach

1 large cucumber

¼ cup shredded carrot

2 teaspoons toasted sesame seeds

For The Dressing:

1 medium avocado, pitted

2 stalks of green onion

1/3 cup chopped cucumber

1/2 teaspoon garlic powder

1/4 teaspoon sea salt

2 tablespoons wasabi powder

2 teaspoons apple cider vinegar

1 tablespoon lime juice

4 tablespoons avocado oil

- Place all the ingredients for dressing in a blender and pulse until smooth, set aside until required.
- Remove each end of cucumber and then spiralized it using a vegetable peeler or spiralizer and place in a bowl.
- Add kale, spinach, and carrots, then drizzle with salad dressing and toss until well coated.
- Garnish with sesame seeds and serve.

Per Serving: Net Carbs: 2.9g; Calories: 200.3; Total Fat: 18.5g; Saturated Fat: 2.3g; Protein: 1.5g; Carbs: 7g; Fiber: 4.1g; Sugar: 2.2g

Percentage of Calories: Total Fat: 83%; Protein: 3%; Carbs: 14%;

Spinach and Artichoke Soup

Serves: 6 / Preparation time: 5 minutes / Cooking time: 30 minutes

14-ounce artichoke hearts, chopped

9-ounce frozen chopped spinach

1 medium white onion, peeled and chopped

2 teaspoons minced garlic

1 teaspoon ground black pepper

3 tablespoons avocado oil

1 teaspoon salt

1 ½ cup coconut cream

4 cups vegetable broth

8-ounce vegan cream cheese

1 cup grated vegan parmesan cheese and more for garnishing

- Place a large pot over medium-high heat, add oil and when hot, add onion and cook for 5 minutes or until tender.
- Then add garlic and continue cooking for 1 minute.
- Add spinach, stir well and cook for 5 to 7 minutes or until spinach is warmed through.
- Season with salt and black pepper, add artichoke hearts and broth and cook for 10 minutes.
- Then turn heat to a low level, stir in coconut cream and cream cheese and stir until well combined.
- Stir in cheese and ladle soup into a bowl.
- Garnish with more cheese and serve.

Per Serving: Net Carbs: 10.8g; Calories: 425.8; Total Fat: 36g; Saturated Fat: 18.5g; Protein: 10.6g; Carbs: 15g; Fiber: 4.2g; Sugar: 4.6g

Percentage of Calories: Total Fat: 76%; Protein: 10%; Carbs: 14%;

Creamy Broccoli Soup

Serves: 6 / Preparation time: 10 minutes / Cooking time: 30 minutes

3 cups chopped celery

3 cups chopped broccoli florets

½ teaspoon onion powder

½ teaspoon garlic pepper

¾ teaspoon salt

½ teaspoon ground black pepper

½ teaspoon red pepper flakes

3 tablespoons avocado oil

1 ½ cups coconut milk, full-fat and unsweetened

2 cups vegetable stock

- Place all the ingredients in a large pot and stir until mixed.
- Place the pot over medium heat and cook for 30 minutes or more until broccoli is tender.
- Then remove the pot from heat and puree the soup using an immersion blender until smooth.
- Ladle soup into bowls and serve.

Per Serving: Net Carbs: 14.6g; Calories: 282.2; Total Fat: 22.8g; Saturated Fat: 6.3g; Protein: 2.1g; Carbs: 17g; Fiber: 2.4g; Sugar: 1.3g

Percentage of Calories: Total Fat: 62%; Protein: 34%; Carbs: 4%;

Kale and Spinach Soup

Serves: 4 / Preparation time: 5 minutes / Cooking time: 10 minutes

For Soup:

8-ounce kale

8-ounce fresh spinach

1 teaspoon salt

2 medium avocados, pitted

¼ teaspoon ground black pepper

3-ounce avocado oil

1 lime, juiced

3 1/3 cups coconut milk, full-fat and unsweetened

1 cup water

For Fried Kale:

3-ounce kale leaves

1 teaspoon minced garlic

½ teaspoon ground black pepper

½ teaspoon ground cardamom

½ teaspoon salt

1 teaspoon avocado oil

- Place a large pot over medium heat, add avocado oil and when hot, add spinach and kale.
- Cook for 3 to 5 minutes or until tender-crisp and then remove the pot from heat.
- Add avocado, salt, and black pepper and then pour in coconut milk and water.
- Puree mixture using an immersion blender until smooth and then stir in lime juice.
- Fry kale and for this, place a skillet pan over high heat, add oil and when hot, add kale and garlic.
- Cook for 2 to 3 minutes or until nicely golden.
- Ladle soup into bowls, top with fried kale and serve.

Per Serving: Net Carbs: 14g; Calories: 865; Total Fat: 86g; Saturated Fat: 36.8g; Protein: 11g; Carbs: 25g; Fiber: 11g; Sugar: 8g

Percentage of Calories: Total Fat: 86%; Protein: 5%; Carbs: 9%;

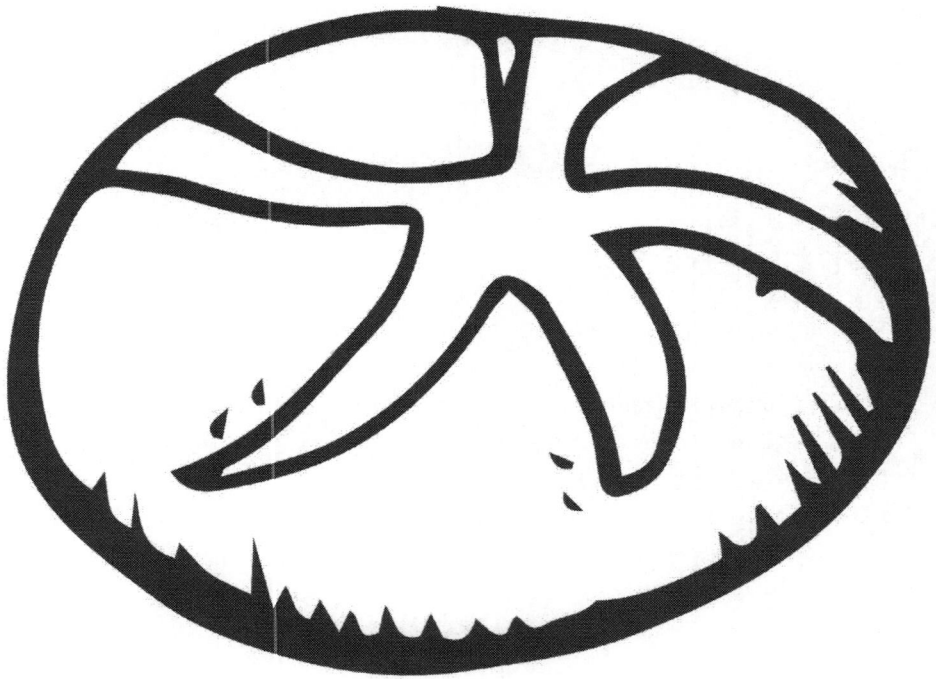

SNACKS AND SIDES RECIPES

Contents

Fried Tempeh 72

Mozzarella Sticks 73

Roasted Cauliflower Steaks 74

Roasted Radishes 75

Mint Matcha Fat Bombs 76

Toasted Coconut Cashews 77

Deviled Avocado 78

Parmesan Fried Eggplant 79

Basil Pesto Zucchini Noodles 80

Zucchini Cakes 81

Garlic Aioli 82

Roasted Bok Choy 83

Guacamole 84

Crackers 85

Coconut Bacon 86

Fried Tempeh

Serves: 3 / Preparation time: 10 minutes / Cooking time: 30 minutes

8-ounce block of tempeh

½ teaspoon smoked salt

1 tablespoon tamari

2 tablespoons maple syrup, sugar-free

2 tablespoons avocado oil

- Set oven to 350 degrees F and let preheat.
- In the meantime, line a baking sheet with parchment paper and set aside until required.
- Whisk together all the ingredients except for tempeh in a bowl and let sit for 5 minutes.
- In the meantime, slice tempeh into ¼ inch thick pieces and then dip into prepared tamari-maple mixture until well coated.
- Place coated tempeh pieces onto prepared baking sheet and place into the oven.
- Bake for 30 minutes until cooked through, flipping halfway through.
- Serve straightaway.

Per Serving: Net Carbs: 1.7g; Calories: 290.5; Total Fat: 21.7g; Saturated Fat: 5.2g; Protein: 15.8g; Carbs: 6.3g; Fiber: 4.6g; Sugar: 2.1g

Percentage of Calories: Total Fat: 67%; Protein: 22%; Carbs: 11%;

Mozzarella Sticks

Serves: 5 / Preparation time: 10 minutes / Cooking time: 25 minutes

10 pieces of hearts of palm

2 tablespoons lupin flour

1/4 teaspoon garlic powder

¼ teaspoon salt

¼ teaspoon ground black pepper

1 teaspoon Italian seasoning

2 tablespoons nutritional yeast

3 tablespoons avocado oil

3 tablespoons water

- Set oven to 375 degrees F and let preheat.
- In the meantime, take a large baking sheet, line with parchment paper and set aside.
- Take a large dish with wide mouth and stir together garlic powder, salt, black pepper, Italian seasoning, yeast, oil and water until combined.
- Drain heart of palm and coat each piece with prepared seasoning mixture on all sides and then place onto prepared baking sheet.
- Place the baking sheet into the oven and bake for 20 to 25 minutes or until nicely golden brown.
- Serve straightaway.

Per Serving: Net Carbs: 2g; Calories: 116.8; Total Fat: 8.9g; Saturated Fat: 1.1g; Protein: 5g; Carbs: 4g; Fiber: 4.5g; Sugar: 0.2g

Percentage of Calories: Total Fat: 69%; Protein: 17%; Carbs: 14%;

Roasted Cauliflower Steaks

Serves: 4 / Preparation time: 5 minutes / Cooking time: 30 minutes

½ of a medium head of cauliflower, sliced into steaks

1 tablespoon grated ginger

1 teaspoon garlic powder

1 teaspoon onion powder

1 teaspoon sea salt

2 tablespoons erythritol sweetener

1 cup tamari sauce

½ cup sesame oil

1 teaspoon toasted sesame seeds, plus more to garnish

- Set oven to 400 degrees F and let preheat.
- In the meantime, whisk together all the ingredients except for salt and cauliflower and pour in a saucepan.
- Place saucepan over medium heat and simmer.
- Then reduce heat to the low level and cook for 3 to 5 minutes or until sauce is reduced to desired thickness.
- Remove pan from heat and baste it on all sides of cauliflower steaks and then season with salt.
- Arrange coated cauliflower steaks on a baking sheet, lined with parchment sheet, and roast for 25 minutes or until cooked.
- Garnish with sesame seeds and serve.

Per Serving: Net Carbs: 2g; Calories: 306.7; Total Fat: 27.3g; Saturated Fat: 4g; Protein: 7.6g; Carbs: 7.6g; Fiber: 2.2g; Sugar: 2.6g

Percentage of Calories: Total Fat: 80%; Protein: 10%; Carbs: 10%;

Roasted Radishes

20 medium radishes, trimmed and quartered

2 green onions, sliced

1 1/2 tablespoon soy sauce

1 1/2 tablespoon roasted peanut oil

1 teaspoon toasted sesame oil

3 teaspoons black sesame seeds

- Set oven to 425 degrees F and let preheat.
- In the meantime, take a large baking sheet and grease with oil.
- Place radish in a large bowl, add peanut oil, toss until well coated and then arrange on prepared baking sheet, cut-side down.
- Place the baking sheet into the oven and bake for 20 minutes or until tender, stirring twice.
- Meanwhile, whisk together soy sauce and sesame oil.
- When radish is roasted, brush radish with sesame oil mixture and continue roasting for 5 to 7 minutes.
- When done, garnish with sesame seeds and green onions and serve.

Per Serving: Net Carbs: 0.5g; Calories: 88.6; Total Fat: 9g; Saturated Fat: 1.5g; Protein: 0.6g; Carbs: 1.1g; Fiber: 0.6g; Sugar: 0.5g

Percentage of Calories: Total Fat: 92%; Protein: 3%; Carbs: 5%;

Mint Matcha Fat Bombs

Serves: 10 / Preparation time: 5 minutes / Cooking time: 30 minutes

3/4 cup hemp seeds

1 teaspoon liquid stevia

1 teaspoon matcha powder

1/2 teaspoon vanilla extract, unsweetened

1/2 teaspoon mint extract, unsweetened

2 tablespoons coconut butter

1/2 cup avocado oil

- Place all ingredients except for coconut butter in a blend and pulse at high speed until smooth.
- Divide mixture between 10 silicon muffin tins.
- Place coconut butter in a heatproof bowl and microwave for 30 seconds or until melted.
- Drizzle melted butter on top of muffin tins in decorative swirls.
- Serve straightaway.

Per Serving: Net Carbs: 1.1g; Calories: 199.6; Total Fat: 20.2g; Saturated Fat: 12.7g; Protein: 4.2g; Carbs: 2.4g; Fiber: 1.3g; Sugar: 0.7g

Percentage of Calories: Total Fat: 87%; Protein: 8%; Carbs: 5%;

Toasted Coconut Cashews

Serves: 20 / Preparation time: 15 minutes / Cooking time: 45 minutes

3 cups cashews, unsalted

1/2 cup toasted coconut flakes

1/2 teaspoon salt

1 tablespoon cinnamon

1 cup monk fruit sweetener, granulated

1 teaspoon vanilla extract, unsweetened

1/4 cup water

- Set oven to 250 degrees F and let preheat.
- Take a large baking sheet, line with parchment paper and set aside.
- Place sweetener in a heatproof bowl, stir in water and microwave for 1 minute or until melted.
- Pour melted sweetener over cashews, stir until evenly coated and then spread on prepared baking sheet in a single layer.
- Place the baking sheet into the oven and bake for 45 minutes or until cashews begin to crystallize.
- Then remove baking sheet from the oven, let cool for 2 minutes, stir and let cool completely.
- Once cashews are cooled, sprinkle with coconut flakes and toss until coated.
- Serve straightaway.

Per Serving: Net Carbs: 1g; Calories: 103; Total Fat: 7g; Saturated Fat: 2g; Protein: 8g; Carbs: 2g; Fiber: 1g; Sugar: 0.3g

Percentage of Calories: Total Fat: 61%; Protein: 31%; Carbs: 8%;

Deviled Avocado

Serves: 4 / Preparation time: 10 minutes / Cooking time: 0 minutes

2 large avocado, pitted

1 teaspoon chopped cilantro

For Sriracha Filling:

1/2 cup and 2 tablespoons mashed avocado

¼ teaspoon salt

1/8 teaspoon ground black pepper

1/8 teaspoon red chili powder

1/8 teaspoon paprika

2 tablespoons Sriracha

4 teaspoons lime juice

2 tablespoons vegan mayonnaise

- Stir together all the ingredients for Sriracha filling until well combined.
- Cut each avocado into half, lengthwise, remove the pit and fill with Sriracha filling.
- Garnish with cilantro and serve.

Per Serving: Net Carbs: 6g; Calories: 420; Total Fat: 36g; Saturated Fat: 5g; Protein: 4g; Carbs: 20g; Fiber: 14g; Sugar: 1g

Percentage of Calories: Total Fat: 77%; Protein: 4%; Carbs: 19%;

Parmesan Fried Eggplant

Serves: 6 / Preparation time: 5 minutes / Cooking time: 30 minutes

1 cup almond flour

1 medium eggplant

¼ cup silken tofu

2 teaspoons garlic powder

1 teaspoon salt, divided

1/2 teaspoon ground black pepper

1 cup grated Parmesan cheese, vegan

1/2 cup avocado oil

- Slice eggplant into 1/3 inch pieces and arrange on a baking sheet, in a single layer, and season with salt.
- Let eggplant sit for 30 minutes and then dry with paper towels.
- Place flour in a shallow dish and stir in garlic, salt, black pepper, and parmesan cheese.
- Place tofu in another dish.
- Place a large skillet pan over medium heat, add 2 tablespoons oil and let heat.
- In the meantime, coat eggplant slice with tofu and then dredge with almond flour mixture.
- Coat remaining eggplant slices in the same manner and add to heated pan in a single layer.
- Cool for 3 to 5 minutes per side or until crispy and nicely browned and then transfer to a plate lined with paper towels.
- Cook remaining eggplant slices, in the same manner, using the remaining oil.
- Serve straightaway.

Per Serving: Net Carbs: 6g; Calories: 376; Total Fat: 32g; Saturated Fat: 11g; Protein: 12g; Carbs: 10g; Fiber: 4g; Sugar: 3g

Percentage of Calories: Total Fat: 77%; Protein: 13%; Carbs: 10%;

Basil Pesto Zucchini Noodles

2 cups basil leaves, fresh

1 large clove of garlic, peeled

1/3 cup toasted pine nuts

¾ teaspoon sea salt

½ teaspoon ground black pepper

1 tablespoon nutritional yeast

1/3 cup olive oil

Zucchini noodles for serving

- Place peeled garlic in a blender and pulse until chopped.
- Then add remaining ingredients except for zucchini noodles and pulse until smooth.
- Tip pesto in a bowl, add zucchini noodles and toss until evenly coated.
- Serve straightaway.

Per Serving: Net Carbs: 3.3g; Calories: 332; Total Fat: 32g; Saturated Fat: 4.7g; Protein: 4.2g; Carbs: 6.6g; Fiber: 3.3g; Sugar: 3g

Percentage of Calories: Total Fat: 87%; Protein: 5%; Carbs: 8%;

Zucchini Cakes

Serves: 2 / Preparation time: 25 minutes / Cooking time: 40 minutes

2 cups grated zucchini

1 tablespoon chopped dill

1/4 teaspoon garlic powder

1/2 teaspoon salt

1/4 cup pea protein powder

1 tablespoon mustard paste

2 tablespoons avocado oil

- Set oven to 350 degrees F and let preheat.
- Place grated zucchini in a large bowl, season with salt, stir well and let rest for 20 minutes.
- Then wrap zucchini in cheesecloth and twist to remove the excess moisture completely.
- Return zucchini into a bowl and add gill, garlic, and mustard and stir until combined.
- Stir in protein powder and shape mixture into four patties.
- Place patties on a parchment lined baking sheet and press lightly to flat patties about ½ inch.
- Place the baking sheet into the oven and bake for 35 to 40 minutes or until nicely browned on all sides, flipping halfway through.
- Serve straightaway.

Per Serving: Net Carbs: 3.8g; Calories: 250; Total Fat: 19g; Saturated Fat: 4g; Protein: 14.1g; Carbs: 5.8g; Fiber: 2g; Sugar: 0.5g

Percentage of Calories: Total Fat: 68%; Protein: 23%; Carbs: 9%;

Garlic Aioli

Serves: 4 / Preparation time: 5 minutes / Cooking time: 0 minutes

3/4 cup vegan mayonnaise

1 ½ teaspoon minced garlic

1/4 teaspoon sea salt

1/4 teaspoon ground black pepper

2 1/2 tablespoons lemon juice

- Place all the ingredients in a bowl and whisk until combined.
- Cover the bowl and chill in the refrigerator for 30 minutes.
- Serve aioli with sliced veggies.

Per Serving: Net Carbs: 0.66g; Calories: 306; Total Fat: 33g; Saturated Fat: 5.3g; Protein: 1.5g; Carbs: 0.76g; Fiber: 0.1g; Sugar: 1g

Percentage of Calories: Total Fat: 97%; Protein: 2%; Carbs: 1%;

Roasted Bok Choy

Serves: 4 / Preparation time: 10 minutes / Cooking time: 20 minutes

1 large head of bok choy

2 teaspoons minced garlic

1 teaspoon sea salt

1/2 teaspoon ground black pepper

1/4 cup avocado oil

- Set oven to 425 degrees F and let preheat.
- In the meantime, cut bok choy into eights, lengthwise, and arrange on a large baking sheet in a single layer, cut side down.
- Drizzle 2 tablespoons oil on bok choy pieces, season with ½ teaspoon salt and ¼ teaspoon black pepper.
- Turn bok choy pieces, then drizzle with remaining oil and season with remaining salt and black pepper.
- Spread bok choy with minced garlic and place baking sheet into the oven.
- Bake for 20 minutes or until its leaves are lightly charred, rotating the pan halfway through.
- Serve straightaway.

Per Serving: Net Carbs: 0.9g; Calories: 137.5; Total Fat: 13.6g; Saturated Fat: 1.6g; Protein: 1.7g; Carbs: 2g; Fiber: 1.1g; Sugar: 1.3g

Percentage of Calories: Total Fat: 89%; Protein: 5%; Carbs: 6%;

Guacamole

Serves: 4 / Preparation time: 10 minutes / Cooking time: 0 minutes

3 avocados, halved and pitted

1 jalapeno pepper, seeds removed and diced

2 Roma tomatoes, diced

3 tablespoons chopped fresh cilantro

1 teaspoon minced garlic

1/2 teaspoon sea salt

1 tablespoon avocado oil

1 lime, juiced

- Scoop the flesh of avocado in a bowl and mash with a fork.
- Then add remaining ingredients and stir well.
- Serve straightaway.

Per Serving: Net Carbs: 1.7g; Calories: 212; Total Fat: 18.2g; Saturated Fat: 2.5g; Protein: 2.6g; Carbs: 9.5g; Fiber: 7.8g; Sugar: 2g

Percentage of Calories: Total Fat: 77%; Protein: 5%; Carbs: 18%;

Crackers

2 tablespoons sunflower seeds

1 cup almond flour

1 tablespoon psyllium husks

3/4 teaspoon sea salt

1 tablespoon avocado oil

2 tablespoons water

- Set oven to 350 degrees F and let preheat.
- In the meantime, place sunflower seeds in a blender, add flour and husks and pulse until well blended.
- Then add oil and water and pulse more until smooth dough comes together.
- Transfer dough on to a parchment paper and press to flatten it.
- Cover dough with another parchment paper and roll into 1/8 to 1/16 inch thickness.
- Then remove the top parchment paper and then cut dough into 1-inch squares using a knife.
- Sprinkle with salt and transfer the dough onto a baking sheet.
- Place the baking sheet into the oven and bake for 10 to 15 minutes or until nicely brown and crispy.
- When done, let crackers cool completely and then serve.

Per Serving: Net Carbs: 3g; Calories: 151; Total Fat: 13g; Saturated Fat: 2g; Protein: 4g; Carbs: 6g; Fiber: 3g; Sugar: 0g

Percentage of Calories: Total Fat: 75%; Protein: 10%; Carbs: 15%;

Coconut Bacon

Serves: 4 / Preparation time: 5 minutes / Cooking time: 25 minutes

3 1/2 cups coconut flakes, unsweetened

1 teaspoon smoked paprika

2 tablespoons liquid smoke

1 tablespoon soy sauce

1 tablespoon maple syrup, sugar-free

1 tablespoon water

- Set oven to 350 degrees F and let preheat.
- Place liquid smoke, soy sauce and maple syrup in a large bowl and whisk until combined.
- Add coconut flakes and toss until evenly coated.
- Then spoon the mixture on a non-stick baking sheet and spread evenly.
- Place the baking sheet into the oven and bake for 20 to 25 minutes, flipping every 5 minutes.
- When done, let coconut bacon cool completely and then dice into bite size pieces.
- Serve straightaway or store in refrigerator for a month.

Per Serving: Net Carbs: 7.5g; Calories: 474.7; Total Fat: 42.2g; Saturated Fat: 40g; Protein: 4.7g; Carbs: 18.9g; Fiber: 11.4g; Sugar: 8.1g

Percentage of Calories: Total Fat: 80%; Protein: 4%; Carbs: 16%;

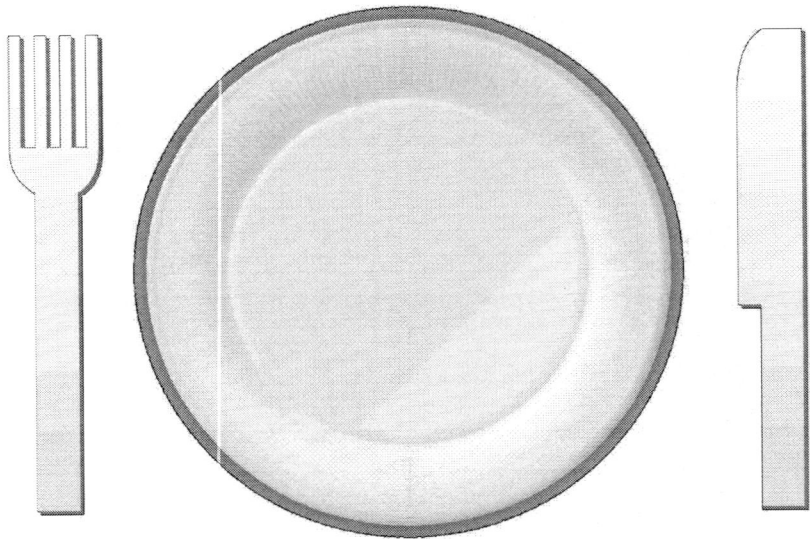

LUNCH RECIPES

Contents

Sloppy Joes 90

Bibimbap 91

Kelp Noodles with Avocado Pesto 92

Falafel 93

Tofu and Shirataki Noodle 94

Roasted Cabbage with Lemon 95

Roasted Eggplant 96

Mashed Garlic Cauliflower 97

Balsamic Glazed Mushrooms 98

Zucchini Noodles with Hemp Pesto 99

Whole Roasted Cauliflower 100

Broccoli Fried Rice 101

Zucchini Noodles with Avocado Sauce 102

Tofu & Cauliflower Rice 103

Peanut Shirataki noodles 104

Sloppy Joes

Serves: 6 / Preparation time: 5 minutes / Cooking time: 45 minutes

1 cup pepitas

1/2 cup hulled hemp seeds

1 cup chopped walnuts

1/2 tablespoon garlic powder

1 teaspoon onion powder

1 tablespoon swerve sweetener

1 tablespoon apple cider vinegar

1 tablespoon prepared mustard

6-ounce tomato paste

2 cups vegetable broth

Lettuce leaves for serving

- Place all the ingredients in a large pot and then place it over medium-low heat.
- Cover the pot and cook for 45 minutes or until broth is absorbed completely, stirring occasionally.
- Serve Sloppy Joes as a lettuce wrap.

Per Serving: Net Carbs: 8.9g; Calories: 382; Total Fat: 30g; Saturated Fat: 18g; Protein: 14.7g; Carbs: 13.5g; Fiber: 4.6g; Sugar: 2.3g

Percentage of Calories: Total Fat: 71%; Protein: 15%; Carbs: 14%;

Bibimbap

Serves: 2 / Preparation time: 10 minutes / Cooking time: 20 minutes

7-ounce tempeh, sliced into squares

1/2 of a medium cucumber, cut into strips

10-ounce cauliflower, riced

6 broccoli florets, cut into spears

1 small red bell pepper, cored and cut in strips

1 medium carrot, grated

15 drops of stevia

2 tablespoon soy sauce, divided

2 tablespoons Sriracha

4 tablespoons apple cider vinegar, divided

1 teaspoon sesame oil

½ cup avocado oil, divided

2 tablespoons sesame seeds

- Whisk together 1 tablespoon soy sauce and 2 tablespoons vinegar in a large bowl, then add tempeh and toss until well coated, set aside for 5 minutes.
- Then place a large skillet over medium heat, add 2 tablespoon avocado oil and when hot, add coated tempeh pieces in a single layer and cook for 5 to 7 minutes until done.
- Cook remaining tempeh in the same manner, using more oil.
- When done, remove tempeh to a plate, add 1 tablespoon avocado oil and then add broccoli, peppers, and carrots.
- Cook for 2 minutes or until vegetables are tender-crisp, covering the pan.
- In the meantime, place another skillet pan over medium heat, add remaining oil and when hot, add cauliflower rice and stir-fry for 5 minutes or until tender.
- When done, divide cauliflower rice evenly between two plates and top with tempeh and vegetables and cucumber.
- Whisk together remaining ingredients except for sesame seeds and pour over tempeh and vegetables.
- Sprinkle with sesame seeds and serve.

Per Serving: Net Carbs: 15.8g; Calories: 912.5; Total Fat: 68g; Saturated Fat: 9.5g; Protein: 27.3g; Carbs: 47.9g; Fiber: 32.1g; Sugar: 17g

Percentage of Calories: Total Fat: 67%; Protein: 12%; Carbs: 21%;

Kelp Noodles with Avocado Pesto

Serves: 1 / Preparation time: 30 minutes / Cooking time: 0 minutes

12-ounce kelp noodles

1 cup fresh baby spinach leaves

1 medium Hass avocado, pitted

1/4 cup fresh basil

1 teaspoon minced garlic

1 teaspoon salt

1/2 cup avocado oil

- Rinse noodles well and then soak them in warm water for 30 minutes.
- In the meantime, place remaining ingredients in a blender and pulse at high speed for 1 to 2 minutes or until smooth.
- Tip the pesto in a bowl.
- Drain the noodles, add to pesto and toss until mixed.
- Serve straightaway.

Per Serving: Net Carbs: 1.3g; Calories: 323.1; Total Fat: 32.7g; Saturated Fat: 18g; Protein: 0.2g; Carbs: 7g; Fiber: 5.7g; Sugar: 0g

Percentage of Calories: Total Fat: 91%; Protein: 0%; Carbs: 9%;

Falafel

Serves: 8 / Preparation time: 10 minutes / Cooking time: 20 minutes

½ cup silken tofu

3 tablespoons coconut flour

1 cup cauliflower florets, pureed

1/2 cup ground slivered almonds

½ teaspoon minced garlic

1 teaspoon salt

1/2 teaspoon cayenne pepper

1 tablespoon ground cumin

1/2 tablespoon ground coriander

2 tablespoons chopped parsley

3 tablespoons avocado oil

- Place pureed cauliflower and almonds in a medium bowl along with remaining ingredients except for oil and stir until mixed.
- Shape mixture into 8 patties, each about 3-inch.
- Place a medium skillet pan over medium heat, add oil and when hot, add four patties to pan.
- Cook for 4 to 5 minutes per side until nicely browned on all sides and then transfer to a plate lined with paper towels.
- Cook remaining falafel in the same manner and serve.

Per Serving: Net Carbs: 5g; Calories: 276; Total Fat: 24g; Saturated Fat: 15g; Protein: 8g; Carbs: 7g; Fiber: 2g; Sugar: 5g

Percentage of Calories: Total Fat: 67%; Protein: 12%; Carbs: 21%;

Tofu and Shirataki Noodle

Serves: 4 / Preparation time: 5 minutes / Cooking time: 25 minutes

14-ounce firm tofu, drained and cut into small cubes

12-ounce shirataki noodles, drained and rinsed

1 bunch of broccoli, chopped into bite-sized pieces

1 medium carrot, shredded

2 cups sliced mushrooms

2 scallions, chopped

1 teaspoon minced garlic

1-inch piece of ginger, peeled and minced

2 teaspoons red pepper flakes

2 tablespoons apple cider vinegar

5 tablespoons soy sauce, divided

1 tablespoon sesame seeds

4 teaspoons avocado oil

1 teaspoon toasted sesame oil

- Place a large skillet over medium-high heat, add 1 tablespoon each of avocado oil and soy sauce, then add tofu and cook for 10 minutes or until browned on all sides.
- When done, transfer tofu to a plate and set aside.
- Then add remaining avocado oil, ginger and garlic to skillet pan and cook for 1 minute or until fragrant.
- Add broccoli, carrots, and mushrooms and cook for 5 minutes or until vegetables are tender-crisp.
- In the meantime, whisk together red pepper flakes, vinegar, remaining soy sauce, and sesame oil until combined.
- Add noodles to sauce along with cooked tofu pieces and scallions and then add to skillet.
- Continue cooking for 5 minutes, stirring frequently.
- Then remove pan from heat, garnish with sesame seeds and serve.

Per Serving: Net Carbs: 5g; Calories: 277; Total Fat: 20.6g; Saturated Fat: 2.4g; Protein: 10.4g; Carbs: 12.5g; Fiber: 7.5g; Sugar: 5.5g

Percentage of Calories: Total Fat: 62%; Protein: 34%; Carbs: 4%;

Roasted Cabbage with Lemon

Serves: 4 / Preparation time: 5 minutes / Cooking time: 30 minutes

1 large head of green cabbage

1 ½ teaspoon sea salt

¾ teaspoon ground black pepper

3 tablespoons lemon juice

3 tablespoons avocado oil

Lemon slices for serving

- Set oven to 450 degrees F and let preheat.
- In the meantime, take a large roasting pan, grease with oil and set aside until required.
- Cut cabbage into 8 wedges and then arrange them in a single layer on prepared pan.
- Whisk together lemon juice and oil, then brush this mixture on both side of cabbage wedge and then season with salt and black pepper.
- Place roasting pan into the oven and bake for 15 minutes or until nicely browned.
- Then carefully turn cabbage wedges and roast for another 10 to 15 minutes or until nicely browned and cooked through.
- Serve cabbage wedges with lemon slices.

Per Serving: Net Carbs: 5.5g; Calories: 172.3; Total Fat: 65g; Saturated Fat: 1.3g; Protein: 2.6g; Carbs: 12.5g; Fiber: 7g; Sugar: 10.4g

Percentage of Calories: Total Fat: 65%; Protein: 64%; Carbs: 29%;

Roasted Eggplant

Serves: 3 / Preparation time: 5 minutes / Cooking time: 10 minutes

1 whole eggplant

1 teaspoon salt

1 teaspoon ground black pepper

4 tablespoons avocado oil

- Set grill and let preheat over high heat.
- Then cut the eggplant into 1-inch thick pieces, then brush with oil and season with salt.
- Place eggplant on heated grill and cook for 3 to 4 minutes per side.
- Then use a cookie cutter to make a small hole in the center of each eggplant slice.
- Serve immediately.

Per Serving: Net Carbs: 5g; Calories: 218; Total Fat: 18.2g; Saturated Fat: 2.2g; Protein: 1.6g; Carbs: 12g; Fiber: 7g; Sugar: 7.1g

Percentage of Calories: Total Fat: 75%; Protein: 3%; Carbs: 22%;

Mashed Garlic Cauliflower

Serves: 4 / Preparation time: 10 minutes / Cooking time: 10 minutes

1 medium head of cauliflower

1 teaspoon minced garlic

1 teaspoon dried thyme

1 teaspoon dried parsley

1 teaspoon dried rosemary

4 tablespoons avocado oil

- Cut cauliflower into florets and rinse well.
- Pour 1-inch water into a large pot, bring to boil and then insert a steamer in it.
- Place cauliflower into the steamer and steam for 6 to 8 minutes.
- In the meantime, place a small saucepan over medium heat, add 1 tablespoon oil and when hot, add garlic and cook for 30 seconds or until fragrant, remove the pan from heat.
- When cauliflower florets are steamed, remove them from the pot, drain them and return to pot.
- Add garlic and remaining ingredients and stir until mixed.
- Mash the mixture using a stick blender until smooth and then serve.

Per Serving: Net Carbs: 4g; Calories: 163.5; Total Fat: 14.3g; Saturated Fat: 1.7g; Protein: 1.6g; Carbs: 6.9g; Fiber: 2.9g; Sugar: 2.8g

Percentage of Calories: Total Fat: 79%; Protein: 4%; Carbs: 17%;

Balsamic Glazed Mushrooms

Serves: 4 / Preparation time: 5 minutes / Cooking time: 3 hours

32 ounces Cremini mushrooms, stem removed

2 teaspoons minced garlic

1/2 teaspoon sea salt

1/4 teaspoon ground black pepper

2 teaspoons stevia

1 tablespoon tamari

2 tablespoons balsamic vinegar

1/4 cup avocado oil

- Place mushrooms in a 4-quart slow cooker along with remaining ingredients and stir until mix.
- Then cover with lid, plug it in and cook for 2 to 3 hours at high heat setting or until cooked through.
- Serve straightaway.

Per Serving: Net Carbs: 12g; Calories: 264; Total Fat: 20g; Saturated Fat: 3g; Protein: 7g; Carbs: 14g; Fiber: 2g; Sugar: 11g

Percentage of Calories: Total Fat: 79%; Protein: 4%; Carbs: 17%;

Zucchini Noodles with Hemp Pesto

Serves: 4 / Preparation time: 5 minutes / Cooking time: 10 minutes

4 medium zucchini, ends removed

2 cups cherry tomatoes, halved

1 teaspoon minced garlic

1/4 teaspoon sea salt

1/4 teaspoon ground black pepper

1 teaspoon dried thyme

4 tablespoons avocado oil

1 cup hemp pesto

- Prepare zucchini noodles by using a vegetable peeler or spiralizer and set aside.
- Place a medium skillet pan over medium heat, add oil and when hot, add remaining ingredients except for pesto.
- Cook for 3 minutes, then add zucchini noodles and hemp pesto and toss gently until mixed.
- Cook for 2 minutes or until heated through and serve.

Per Serving: Net Carbs: 2g; Calories: 431.5; Total Fat: 39.7g; Saturated Fat: 4.3g; Protein: 6.5g; Carbs: 13g; Fiber: 4.4g; Sugar: 7.2g

Percentage of Calories: Total Fat: 83%; Protein: 6%; Carbs: 12%;

Whole Roasted Cauliflower

Serves: 4 / Preparation time: 15 minutes / Cooking time: 25 minutes

1 medium whole cauliflower head, bottom removed
5 tomatoes, diced
2 medium white onions, peeled and diced
1 teaspoon grated ginger
1 teaspoon minced garlic
1/2 cup cashews, soaked in almond milk
1 ½ teaspoon salt
1 teaspoon red chili powder

1/2 teaspoon cumin seeds
1 bay leaf
1/2 teaspoon turmeric powder
1 teaspoon coriander powder
1/2 teaspoon garam masala
4 tablespoons avocado oil
1 teaspoon roasted sesame seeds
1 tablespoon cilantro
2 cups water, hot

- Plug in instant pot, press 'saute' button and when hot, add oil, bay leaf and cumin and cook for 2 minutes or until sizzles.
- Then add onion, garlic, ginger, and salt and cook for 5 minutes or until softened.
- Add salt, red chili powder, cumin, turmeric, coriander powder, and garam masala and continue cooking for 2 minutes.
- Then add tomatoes, stir well and cook for 3 to 5 minutes or until oil separates.
- Add cashews and almond milk, puree the mixture using an immersion blender until smooth.
- Stir in water until combined and transfer sauce to a bowl, set aside until required.
- Insert trivet stand into the instant pot, pour in 1 cup water and place cauliflower on the stand.
- Press cancel, seal instant pot and cook for 0 minutes at high pressure.
- When timer beeps, do quick pressure release, then transfer cauliflower to a roasting pan and let cool for 10 minutes.
- Meanwhile, switch on the broiler and let preheat.
- Pour half of the prepared sauce over cauliflower and then broil for 3 to 5 minutes.
- Garnish with sesame seeds and cilantro and serve.

Per Serving: Net Carbs: 7.6g; Calories: 276; Total Fat: 21.5g; Saturated Fat: 2.6g; Protein: 3.4g; Carbs: 17.2g; Fiber: 9.6g; Sugar: 7g
Percentage of Calories: Total Fat: 70%; Protein: 5%; Carbs: 25%;

Broccoli Fried Rice

Serves: 4 / Preparation time: 5 minutes / Cooking time: 5 minutes

4 cups riced broccoli

½ teaspoon grated ginger

1 tablespoon minced garlic

½ teaspoon salt

1 tablespoon coconut aminos

½ tablespoon lime juice and more for serving

1 ½ teaspoon toasted sesame oil

2 tablespoons avocado oil

4 tablespoons chopped cilantro

- Place a medium skillet pan over medium heat, add avocado oil and when hot, add broccoli rice and garlic and cook for 1 minute.
- Then add salt, coconut aminos, and sesame oil and continue cooking for 2 minutes or until broccoli is tender-crisp.
- Remove pan from heat, stir ginger into the broccoli and then garnish with cilantro.
- Serve straightaway.

Per Serving: Net Carbs: 0.4g; Calories: 105.2; Total Fat: 8.4g; Saturated Fat: 1g; Protein: 3.7g; Carbs: 3.4g; Fiber: 3g; Sugar: 1g

Percentage of Calories: Total Fat: 72%; Protein: 14%; Carbs: 14%;

Zucchini Noodles with Avocado Sauce

Serves: 2 / Preparation time: 10 minutes / Cooking time: 0 minutes

4 tablespoons pine nuts

1 medium zucchini, ends removed

12 sliced of cherry tomatoes

1 medium avocado, pitted

1 1/4 cup basil

2 tablespoons lemon juice

1/3 cup water

- Prepare zucchini using a vegetable peeler or spiralizer.
- Place remaining ingredients in a blender, except for tomatoes, and pulse at high speed until smooth.
- Tip the sauce in a bowl, add zucchini noodles and tomatoes and toss until well coated.
- Serve straightaway.

Per Serving: Net Carbs: 9g; Calories: 233; Total Fat: 29.8g; Saturated Fat: 3.1g; Protein: 6.8g; Carbs: 18.7g; Fiber: 9.7g; Sugar: 6.5g

Percentage of Calories: Total Fat: 73%; Protein: 7%; Carbs: 20%;

Tofu & Cauliflower Rice

Serves: 8 / Preparation time: 5 minutes / Cooking time: 45 minutes

14-ounce extra-firm tofu, pressed and drained

24 ounce frozen riced cauliflower

1 1/2 cups diced carrot

10 ounce chopped scallion

1/3 cup grated ginger

1/4 cup minced garlic

1 ½ teaspoon salt

2 tablespoons soy sauce

2 tablespoons sesame oil, divided

6 tablespoons avocado oil

- Place a large skillet pan over medium-high heat, add sesame oil and when hot, add tofu.
- Scramble tofu with a potato masher and cook for 10 to 15 minutes or until browned, stirring frequently.
- In the meantime, place another large skillet over medium-high heat, add 2 tablespoons avocado oil and when hot, add ginger, garlic, and carrot and cook for 10 minutes or until tender.
- Add 2 tablespoons oil, cauliflower, and scallion and continue cooking for 10 to 15 minutes or until heated through.
- Then add tofu, salt, soy sauce, and remaining oil and toss until mixed.
- Serve straightaway.

Per Serving: Net Carbs: 9.5g; Calories: 336; Total Fat: 25.4g; Saturated Fat: 3.1g; Protein: 10.1g; Carbs: 16.8g; Fiber: 7.3g; Sugar: 7.2g

Percentage of Calories: Total Fat: 68%; Protein: 12%; Carbs: 20%;

Peanut Shirataki noodles

Serves: 1 / Preparation time: 5 minutes / Cooking time: 10 minutes

For Peanut Sauce:

1/8 teaspoon garlic powder

1/8 teaspoon grated ginger

1/4 teaspoon ground black pepper

1 teaspoon swerve sweetener

1 tablespoon soy sauce

1 teaspoon apple cider vinegar

1/4 teaspoon sesame oil

2 tablespoons peanut butter

1 tablespoon water

For Noodles:

8 ounces shirataki spaghetti

6 ounce chopped scallion

Peanuts for garnishing

- Stir together all the ingredients for sauce in a bowl and let sit for 30 minutes.
- Then drain and rinse spaghetti and pat dry.
- Place a medium skillet pan over medium-low heat, add noodles and cook for 2 to 3 minutes or until dry.
- Add scallion and cook for 2 to 3 minutes or until heated through.
- Add prepared peanut sauce and stir well until spaghetti is evenly coated with sauce.
- Garnish with peanuts and serve.

Per Serving: Net Carbs: 4g; Calories: 153.5; Total Fat: 11.5g; Saturated Fat: 3g; Protein: 4.5g; Carbs: 8g; Fiber: 4g; Sugar: 1g

Percentage of Calories: Total Fat: 67%; Protein: 12%; Carbs: 21%;

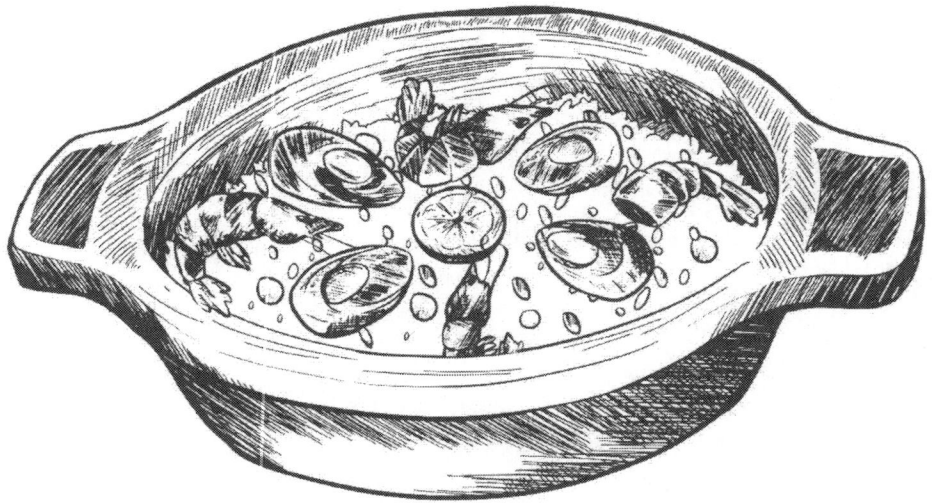

DINNER RECIPES

Contents

Cauliflower Tofu Tacos 108

Zucchini Tomato Pesto 109

Shirataki Noodles with Almond Butter Sauce 110

Cauliflower Fried Rice 111

Tofu in Purgatory 112

Kale & Crispy Coconut Tempeh 113

Zucchini Lasagna 114

Roasted Lemon Vegetables 115

Zucchini Pasta 116

Portobello Mushroom "Tacos" 117

Cauliflower Pizza Crust 118

Cauliflower Rice Pilaf 119

Hemp Seed Lettuce Wraps 120

Walnut Chili 121

Spinach Artichoke Pizza 122

Cauliflower Tofu Tacos

Serves: 6 / Preparation time: 5 minutes / Cooking time: 30 minutes

14-ounce extra-firm tofu, pressed and drained
1/2 pound cremini mushrooms, sliced
1 large head of cauliflower, cut into florets
2 medium orange bell peppers, cored and sliced
1 large white onion, peeled and diced
8 tablespoons avocado oil, divided
1/2 teaspoon garlic powder
2 ½ teaspoons sea salt

2 teaspoons ground black pepper
1/2 teaspoon cumin
1 teaspoon paprika
1 teaspoon red chili powder
1/2 teaspoon red chili flakes
1 tablespoon taco seasoning
2 teaspoons vegan Worcestershire sauce
1 tablespoon apple cider vinegar
1 tablespoon tomato paste
1/4 cup fresh cilantro for garnishing

- Set oven to 400 degrees F and let preheat.
- In the meantime, take a large baking tray, line with parchment paper and arrange mushrooms, cauliflower, and peppers.
- Season with 1 ½ teaspoon salt and 1 teaspoon black pepper, drizzle with 4 tablespoons oil and toss until coated.
- Place the baking sheet into the oven and bake for 25 to 30 minutes or until vegetables are tender and nicely browned.
- In the meantime, place a large skillet over medium heat, add remaining oil and onion and cook for 5 minutes or until tender.
- Add tofu into the pan and scramble it using a potato masher.
- Add remaining ingredients, stir until well coated and cook for 10 minutes, stirring occasionally.
- When vegetables are roasted, transfer them to skillet pan and stir until combined.
- Garnish with cilantro and serve with favorite taco topping.

Per Serving: Net Carbs: 2g; Calories: 265.2; Total Fat: 20g; Saturated Fat: 2.6g; Protein: 7.3g; Carbs: 14g; Fiber: 4.2g; Sugar: 6.5g
Percentage of Calories: Total Fat: 68%; Protein: 11%; Carbs: 21%;

Zucchini Tomato Pesto

Serves: 6 / Preparation time: 10 minutes / Cooking time: 35 minutes

For Pesto Sauce:

1 tablespoon pumpkin seeds

1 cup fresh basil leaves

1 teaspoon minced garlic

1 teaspoon sea salt

½ teaspoon ground black pepper

1/4 cup avocado oil

1 tablespoon water

For Vegetables:

3 medium zucchini, sliced

8 medium cherry tomatoes, sliced

2 small red onions, peeled and sliced

1 teaspoon sea salt

½ teaspoon ground black pepper

1/4 teaspoon Italian seasoning

2 tablespoons avocado oil

- Set oven to 350 degrees F and let preheat.
- In the meantime, place all the ingredients of pesto in a blender and pulse until smooth, set aside until required.
- Prepare vegetables and for this, place a skillet pan over medium heat, add oil and when hot, layer vegetables in it, first some zucchini slices, then tomato slices, onion slices and creating more layers in the same manner until all vegetables are used up.
- Brush each vegetable layer with prepared pesto, then season with salt, black pepper, and Italian seasoning and cover pan with parchment paper.
- Place pan into the oven and bake for 30 to 35 minutes or until vegetables are soft.
- Serve straightaway.

Per Serving: Net Carbs: 7.1g; Calories: 183; Total Fat: 14.6g; Saturated Fat: 1.8g; Protein: 2.3g; Carbs: 10.5g; Fiber: 3.4g; Sugar: 5.7g

Percentage of Calories: Total Fat: 72%; Protein: 5%; Carbs: 23%;

Shirataki Noodles with Almond Butter Sauce

Serves: 6 / Preparation time: 5 minutes / Cooking time: 10 minutes

12-ounce Shirataki noodles

3.5-ounce broccoli

¼ of a medium cabbage, shredded

1 teaspoon minced garlic

2 tablespoons avocado oil

1 small carrot, diced

2 tablespoons coconut aminos

2 teaspoons sriracha sauce

1 tablespoon almond butter

- Place a large saucepan over medium heat, add oil and when hot, add onion and garlic.
- Cook for 3 to 5 minutes or until tender, then add broccoli, and cabbage and cook for 3 to 5 minutes or until tender crisp.
- Drain noodles, rinse well and then add to vegetables.
- Add remaining ingredients and toss until well mixed.
- Serve straightaway.

Per Serving: Net Carbs: 1.6g; Calories: 79.2; Total Fat: 5.8g; Saturated Fat: 0.6g; Protein: 1.4g; Carbs: 5.1g; Fiber: 3.5g; Sugar: 1.5g

Percentage of Calories: Total Fat: 67%; Protein: 7%; Carbs: 26%;

Cauliflower Fried Rice

Serves: 4 / Preparation time: 5 minutes / Cooking time: 15 minutes

1 pound firm tofu, pressed and drained

1 medium head of cauliflower, riced

1 cup sliced carrot

1/4 cup thinly sliced green onions

1 ½ teaspoon minced garlic

1 tablespoon minced ginger

3 tablespoons soy sauce

3 tablespoons cashews

2 tablespoons sesame oil, divided

1 tablespoon avocado oil

Sesame seeds for garnishing

- Place a large skillet pan over medium heat, add sesame oil and when hot, add ginger and garlic.
- Cook for 1 minute or until fragrant, then add tofu and crumble with a potato masher.
- Stir well and stir-fry for 5 minutes or until tofu is nicely golden brown and cooked through.
- Transfer tofu to a bowl and add oil into the pan and when hot, add carrots and cook for 2 minutes or until tender.
- Add cauliflower rice, stir well until mix thoroughly and cook for 5 to 8 minutes or until tender.
- Add tofu and remaining ingredients and remove the pan from heat.
- Garnish with sesame seeds and serve.

Per Serving: Net Carbs: 5.5g; Calories: 211.7; Total Fat: 14.8g; Saturated Fat: 2g; Protein: 10g; Carbs: 9.5g; Fiber: 4g; Sugar: 4.9g

Percentage of Calories: Total Fat: 63%; Protein: 19%; Carbs: 18%;

Tofu in Purgatory

Serves: 2 / Preparation time: 5 minutes / Cooking time: 20 minutes

12-ounce firm tofu, pressed and drained

3 1/3 cups diced tomatoes

2 teaspoons minced garlic

1 teaspoon salt

1 teaspoon swerve sweetener

½ teaspoon ground black pepper

1/2 teaspoon red chili flakes

1 teaspoon dried thyme

1 teaspoon dried parsley

2 tablespoons avocado oil

- Place a large skillet pan over medium heat, add oil and when hot, add garlic and cook for 1 minute or until fragrant.
- Then add tomatoes, salt, black pepper, sweetener, red chili flakes, thyme, and parsley and stir until mixed.
- Simmer mixture for 5 minutes, then add tofu and simmer at medium-low heat for 15 minutes or until sauce is slightly thickened and tofu is heated through.
- Serve straightaway.

Per Serving: Net Carbs: 10.3g; Calories: 287; Total Fat: 61g; Saturated Fat: 2.35g; Protein: 13.6g; Carbs: 14.3g; Fiber: 4.2g; Sugar: 7.1g

Percentage of Calories: Total Fat: 61%; Protein: 19%; Carbs: 20%;

Kale & Crispy Coconut Tempeh

Serves: 4 / Preparation time: 5 minutes / Cooking time: 20 minutes

1 package of tempeh, cut into small pieces

1 bunch of kale, chopped

3 sliced green onions, divided

2-inch piece of lemongrass, diced

1 Thai green chili

¼ cup cilantro leaves, divided

2 limes

1 tablespoon grated ginger

2 teaspoons salt

½ teaspoon ground black pepper

1 teaspoon ground coriander

1 teaspoon soy sauce

6 tablespoons avocado oil, divided

1/2 cup coconut milk, unsweetened and full-fat

1 lime, juiced and zested

1 teaspoon hemp seeds

- Place kale, green parts of onions and half of the cilantro in a large bowl, add ½ teaspoon salt, ¼ teaspoon black pepper, 2 tablespoons oil and lime juice, toss until combined and then massage kale leaves for 30 seconds until softened, set aside until required.
- Add lemongrass, half of white part of the onion, green chili, chili, remaining cilantro, coriander and ½ teaspoon salt, lime zest in a food processor and pulse until chopped and chunky paste comes together.
- Tip the mixture in a bowl, add soy sauce and taste to adjust seasoning.
- Place a large skillet pan over medium heat, add 2 tablespoons oil and when hot, add remaining onion and cook for 1 minute.
- Add tempeh, season with salt and black pepper, toss until mixed and cook for 8 to 10 minutes or until nicely brown and crispy.
- Divide the prepared kale salad between four plates, top with cooked tempeh and drizzle with coconut dressing.
- Garnish with hemp seeds and serve straightaway.

Per Serving: Net Carbs: 8.5g; Calories: 406.2; Total Fat: 20.8g; Saturated Fat: 5.1g; Protein: 19.3g; Carbs: 15.2g; Fiber: 6.7g; Sugar: 4.2g

Percentage of Calories: Total Fat: 66%; Protein: 19%; Carbs: 15%;

Zucchini Lasagna

Serves: 9 / Preparation time: 10 minutes / Cooking time: 60 minutes

For Lasagna:

3 medium zucchini, thinly sliced

28-ounce marinara sauce, organic and unsweetened

½ cup grated vegan parmesan cheese

For Cheese Filling:

16-ounces extra firm tofu, drained and pressed

1 teaspoon sea salt

¾ teaspoon ground black pepper

1/2 cup fresh basil

2 teaspoons dried oregano

2 tablespoons lemon juice

2 tablespoons nutritional yeast

1 tablespoon avocado oil

1/4 cup grated vegan parmesan cheese

1/2 cup water

- Set oven to 375 degrees F and let preheat.
- Place tofu in a bowl, crumble it with a potato masher and then add to a food processor or blender.
- Add remaining ingredients for cheese filling and pulse until smooth and well combined.
- Take a 9 by 13-inch baking dish, spread 1 cup marinara sauce in the bottom of dish, top with some zucchini slices in a single layer and then spread with some of the cheese filling in a thin layer.
- Create two layers in the same manner, using zucchini slices, marinara sauce, and cheese filling and sprinkle cheese on top.
- Cover baking dish with foil and bake for 45 minutes.
- Then uncover baking dish and continue baking for 15 minutes or until top is nicely brown.
- Slice and serve lasagna straightaway.

Per Serving: Net Carbs: 5g; Calories: 364.8; Total Fat: 34g; Saturated Fat: 5.4g; Protein: 4.7g; Carbs: 10g; Fiber: 5g; Sugar: 3g

Percentage of Calories: Total Fat: 84%; Protein: 5%; Carbs: 11%;

Roasted Lemon Vegetables

Serves: 4 / Preparation time: 10 minutes / Cooking time: 30 minutes

1 medium head of cauliflower, cut into florets

3 medium green bell peppers, sliced

1 medium red onion, peeled and sliced

1/2 cup basil leaves

1 teaspoon sea salt

½ teaspoon ground black pepper

1/2 teaspoon turmeric

1 large lemon, juiced and zested

4 tablespoons avocado oil

- Set oven to 400 degrees F and let preheat.
- In the meantime, blend together salt, black pepper, turmeric, lemon juice, and zest and oil until smooth.
- Arrange all vegetables on a large parchment lined baking tray, then pour prepared lemon sauce on it and stir until well coated.
- Cover vegetables in baking tray with aluminum foil and cook in the oven for 25 to 30 minutes or until tender.
- Serve straightaway.

Per Serving: Net Carbs: 5.9g; Calories: 186; Total Fat: 14.5; Saturated Fat: 1.8g; Protein: 3.2; Carbs: 10.7g; Fiber: 4.8g; Sugar: 6.1g

Percentage of Calories: Total Fat: 70%; Protein: 7%; Carbs: 23%;

Zucchini Pasta

Serves: 4 / Preparation time: 5 minutes / Cooking time: 10 minutes

5 large zucchini, spiralized

1-pint cherry tomatoes, halved

1/2 cup fresh basil

1 medium red onion, peeled and sliced

2 teaspoons minced garlic

1 teaspoon salt

½ teaspoon ground black pepper

1/2 teaspoon crushed red pepper

1/3 cup avocado oil

¼ cup grated parmesan cheese

- Place a large pot over medium heat, add oil and when hot, add onion and garlic and cook for 3 minutes or until fragrant.
- Add zucchini noodles, season with salt and black pepper and continue cooking for 2 minutes, covering the pot.
- Then add tomatoes and cook for 4 to 5 minutes, stirring every 30 seconds and toss until well mixed.
- Add remaining ingredients, stir until combined and then divide pasta evenly between serving plates.
- Serve straightaway.

Per Serving: Net Carbs: 10.8g; Calories: 276.2; Total Fat: 20.8g; Saturated Fat: 3.4g; Protein: 5.5g; Carbs: 15.8g; Fiber: 5g; Sugar: 6.6g

Percentage of Calories: Total Fat: 68%; Protein: 23%; Carbs: 9%;

Portobello Mushroom "Tacos"

Serves: 6 / Preparation time: 20 minutes / Cooking time: 10 minutes

1 pound portobello mushrooms, stem removed

1 teaspoon onion powder

1/4 cup harissa

1 teaspoon ground cumin

3 tablespoons avocado oil, divided

6 collard green leaves, stem removed

1 cup guacamole

Cashew cream for topping

- Whisk together onion powder, harissa, cumin and avocado oil in a bowl and then brush this mixture on mushroom and marinate for 15 minutes.
- In the meantime, prepare guacamole.
- Then place a large skillet pan over medium-high heat, add 1 ½ tablespoon oil and then add marinated mushrooms.
- Cook for 3 minutes per side or until nicely brown and then slice.
- Fill collard greens with few slices of mushroom, top with guacamole and cashew cream and serve.

Per Serving: Net Carbs: 10g; Calories: 445.6; Total Fat: 34.4g; Saturated Fat: 5g; Protein: 10g; Carbs: 24g; Fiber: 14g; Sugar: 5.6g

Percentage of Calories: Total Fat: 69%; Protein: 10%; Carbs: 21%;

Cauliflower Pizza Crust

Serves: 4 / Preparation time: 10 minutes / Cooking time: 30 minutes

6 cups cauliflower florets

1 cup ground flax seeds

1 teaspoon garlic powder

1 teaspoon onion powder

1 teaspoon salt

½ teaspoon ground black pepper

1/2 cup nutritional yeast

2 teaspoons basil

2 teaspoons oregano

2 tablespoons avocado oil

- Set oven to 400 degrees F and let preheat.
- In the meantime, place cauliflower florets in a heatproof bowl, cover with plastic wrap and microwave for 3 to 5 minutes or until steamed and tender.
- Then cool cauliflower, wrap in a cheesecloth and twist well to squeeze out most of the moisture.
- Transfer cauliflower in a food processor, add remaining ingredients and pulse at high speed until well combined.
- Take a pizza pan, grease with oil and spread ¼ of the mixture into ¼ inch thick layer.
- Place the pizza pan into the oven and bake for 10 minutes, then flip crust and continue cooking for another 10 minutes.
- Scatter favorite topping on top, bake for another 3 to 5 minutes and serve.

Per Serving: Net Carbs: 2g; Calories: 392; Total Fat: 28g; Saturated Fat: 3g; Protein: 13g; Carbs: 21g; Fiber: 15g; Sugar: 3g

Percentage of Calories: Total Fat: 64%; Protein: 14%; Carbs: 22%;

Cauliflower Rice Pilaf

Serves: 4 / Preparation time: 5 minutes / Cooking time: 5 minutes

2 cups cauliflower rice

1/2 cup hemp seeds

4 pitted dates, chopped

1 teaspoon salt

½ teaspoon ground black pepper

1/2 teaspoon turmeric

1/2 teaspoon cumin

1/2 cup vegetable broth

1/4 cup sliced almonds

- Place cauliflower rice in a pan along with remaining ingredients, except for almonds, and stir well.
- Place pan over medium heat and cook for 5 minutes or more until all liquid is absorbed.
- Garnish with sliced almonds and serve.

Per Serving: Net Carbs: 5g; Calories: 198; Total Fat: 14g; Saturated Fat: 1g; Protein: 11g; Carbs: 7g; Fiber: 2g; Sugar: 4g

Percentage of Calories: Total Fat: 64%; Protein: 22%; Carbs: 14%;

Hemp Seed Lettuce Wraps

Serves: 4 / Preparation time: 1 hour and 5 minutes / Cooking time: 0 minutes

For the Sauce:

1 tablespoon minced ginger

1 tablespoon stevia

2 tablespoons soy sauce

2 tablespoons apple cider vinegar

1 teaspoon sesame oil

For Filling:

1/2 cup chopped cucumber

1/4 cup chopped carrots

2 dates, chopped

1 cup chopped walnuts

1/2 cup hemp seeds

Lettuce leaves for serving

- Stir together all the ingredients for the sauce until combined.
- Then add ingredients for the filling except for lettuce, stir well and chill in the refrigerator for 1 hour.
- Then fill the mixture on lettuce leaves and serve.

Per Serving: Net Carbs: 10g; Calories: 387; Total Fat: 31g; Saturated Fat: 2g; Protein: 14g; Carbs: 13g; Fiber: 3g; Sugar: 6g

Percentage of Calories: Total Fat: 72%; Protein: 15%; Carbs: 13%;

Walnut Chili

Serves: 6 / Preparation time: 5 minutes / Cooking time: 35 minutes

2 1/2 cups soy meat, crumbled

2 medium zucchini, diced

8-ounce cremini mushrooms

2 medium green bell peppers, diced

15 ounce diced tomatoes

5 stalks of celery, diced

1 teaspoon minced garlic

1 teaspoon salt

½ teaspoon ground black pepper

1 1/2 teaspoon ground cinnamon

2 teaspoons red chili powder

4 teaspoons ground cumin

1 ½ teaspoon smoked paprika

2 peppers chipotle pepper in adobo sauce, minced

1 tablespoon cocoa powder, unsweetened

1 cup walnuts, minced

1 1/2 tablespoon tomato paste

4 tablespoons avocado Oil

1/2 cup coconut milk, full-fat

3 cups water

1 medium avocado, pitted

1/2 cup grated parmesan cheese

- Place a large pot over medium heat, add oil and when hot, add celery and cook for 4 minutes or until tender.
- Then add garlic, paprika, cumin, and cinnamon and cook for 2 minutes or until fragrant.
- Add zucchini, mushrooms, and pepper and continue cooking for 5 minutes.
- Add remaining ingredients except for topping and cook for 20 to 25 minutes or until vegetables are tender.
- Top with avocado slices and cheese and serve.

Per Serving: Net Carbs: 2g; Calories: 467.3; Total Fat: 35.8g; Saturated Fat: 9.4g; Protein: 19.8g; Carbs: 16.3g; Fiber: 11.8g; Sugar: 6.4g

Percentage of Calories: Total Fat: 69%; Protein: 17%; Carbs: 14%;

Spinach Artichoke Pizza

Serves: 6 / Preparation time: 5 minutes / Cooking time: 15 minutes

1 cauliflower pizza crust

1 cup chopped spinach

1 cup artichoke hearts, chopped

1-ounce olives, chopped

2 tablespoons avocado oil

3 tablespoons nutritional yeast

1/4 cup shredded vegan parmesan cheese

- Set oven to 350 degrees F and let preheat.
- In the meantime, place pizza crust on a parchment-lined baking sheet.
- Stir together remaining ingredients and top evenly on the crust.
- Place the baking sheet into the oven and bake for 12 to 15 minutes or until spinach mixture is heated through and cheese melts.
- Slice and serve.

Per Serving: Net Carbs: 8.8g; Calories: 230; Total Fat: 15.8g; Saturated Fat: 2.5g; Protein: 8.6g; Carbs: 13.2g; Fiber: 4.4g; Sugar: 1g

Percentage of Calories: Total Fat: 62%; Protein: 15%; Carbs: 23%;

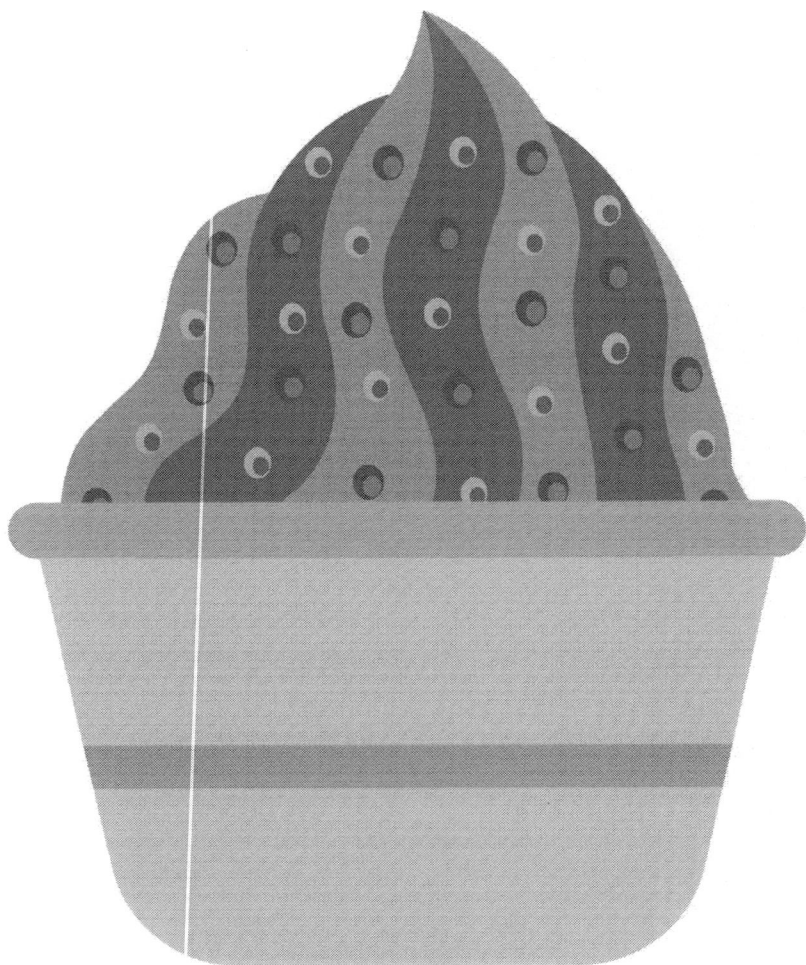

DESSERT RECIPES

Contents

Coconut Dulce De Leche 126
Chocolate Fondue 127
Almond Avocado Pudding.. 128
Strawberry Chia Pudding 129
Avocado Chocolate Mousse... 130
Cinnamon Roll Mug Cake 131
Chocolate Avocado Ice Cream 132
Coconut Fat Bombs 133
Almond Fat Bombs... 134
Chocolate Peppermint Fat Bombs 135
Chocolate Fudge 136
Chocolate Peppermint Chia Pudding 137
Almond Cookies 138
Chocolate Almond Butter Cupcakes 139
Red Velvet Cupcakes.. 140

Coconut Dulce De Leche

Serves: 4 / Preparation time: 15 minutes / Cooking time: 25 minutes

¼ teaspoon salt

¼ cup and 1 tablespoon (60g) swerve sweetener, granulated

28-ounce coconut milk, unsweetened and full-fat

- Place a large saucepan over medium-high heat, add all the ingredients and stir well.
- Cook for 5 minutes and bring the mixture to boil.
- Then turn heat to medium level and continue cooking for 15 to 20 minutes, whisking continuously or until Dulce De Leche have caramel-like consistency and golden color.
- Remove pan from heat, cool for 10 minutes and then transfer to a heat-safe jar and cool completely in the refrigerator.
- Serve straightaway or cover container with lid to store in refrigerator.

Per Serving: Net Carbs: 0.5g; Calories: 35.5; Total Fat: 3.5g; Saturated Fat: 3.3g; Protein: 0.36g; Carbs: 0.7g; Fiber: 0.2g; Sugar: 0.45g

Percentage of Calories: Total Fat: 88%; Protein: 4%; Carbs: 8%;

Chocolate Fondue

Serves: 4 / Preparation time: 5 minutes / Cooking time: 5 minutes

2-ounce dark chocolate, unsweetened

1/8 teaspoon salt

½ teaspoon stevia

1 teaspoon vanilla extract, unsweetened

1/2 cup coconut milk, full-fat

- Place chocolate, salt, vanilla and milk in a heatproof bowl and microwave for 30 seconds.
- Stir until smooth and then slowly stir in stevia, if the mixture is getting hard, microwave for 10 seconds.
- Serve straightaway.

Per Serving: Net Carbs: 3g; Calories: 102; Total Fat: 10.2g; Saturated Fat: 2g; Protein: 2.1g; Carbs: 4.9g; Fiber: 1.9g; Sugar: 1.2g

Percentage of Calories: Total Fat: 77%; Protein: 7%; Carbs: 16%;

Almond Avocado Pudding

Serves: 3 / Preparation time: 5 hours and 10 minutes / Cooking time: 0 minutes

1 medium avocado, peeled and pitted

3 tablespoons swerve sweetener

3 tablespoons cocoa powder, unsweetened

1 teaspoon vanilla extract, unsweetened

1 teaspoon almond extract, unsweetened

1 1/2 cups almond milk, unsweetened and full-fat

1/2 cup coconut cream, unsweetened and full-fat

Coconut flakes for garnishing

- Place all the ingredients in a food processor or blender, except for coconut flakes, and pulse at high speed for 1 minute or more until smooth.
- Divide the mixture evenly between three bowls, cover them and refrigerator for 5 hours or more until chilled.
- Garnish pudding with coconut flakes and serve.

Per Serving: Net Carbs: 4g; Calories: 288; Total Fat: 25g; Saturated Fat: 17g; Protein: 20g; Carbs: 12g; Fiber: 8g; Sugar: 3g

Percentage of Calories: Total Fat: 63%; Protein: 23%; Carbs: 14%;

Strawberry Chia Pudding

Serves: 1 / Preparation time: 4 hours and 5 minutes / Cooking time: 0 minutes

2 strawberries, diced small

1 ½ tablespoons chia seeds

1/2 teaspoon matcha powder

1 teaspoon Stevia

3/4 cup coconut milk, full-fat and unsweetened

- Place all the ingredients except for berries in a bowl and cover with lid.
- Shake the bowl well for 10 seconds and then pour mixture into a glass.
- Chill glass in refrigerator for 4 hours, then top with berries and serve.

Per Serving: Net Carbs: 2g; Calories: 441; Total Fat: 37g; Saturated Fat: 4g; Protein: 7g; Carbs: 20g; Fiber: 13g; Sugar: 5g

Percentage of Calories: Total Fat: 75%; Protein: 7%; Carbs: 18%;

Avocado Chocolate Mousse

Serves: 4 / Preparation time: 2 hours and 5 minutes / Cooking time: 1 minute

2 large avocados, pitted

½ cup and 2 tablespoons organic chocolate chips, semi-sweet

3 tablespoons cocoa powder, unsweetened

1/8 teaspoon salt

3 teaspoons stevia

1 teaspoon vanilla extract, unsweetened

1/4 cup almond milk, unsweetened

- Place chocolate chips in a heatproof bowl and microwave for 15 seconds or more until chocolate melts.
- Stir until smooth and let cool until barely warm.
- Then scoop the flesh of avocado in a blender, add remaining ingredients along with melted chocolate and blend at high speed until smooth and creamy.
- Tip mousse into a bowl and let chill in the refrigerator for 2 hours or more before serving.

Per Serving: Net Carbs: 5g; Calories: 216.2; Total Fat: 17.3g; Saturated Fat: 8g; Protein: 26g; Carbs: 13g; Fiber: 8g; Sugar: 4g

Percentage of Calories: Total Fat: 72%; Protein: 4%; Carbs: 24%;

Cinnamon Roll Mug Cake

Serves: 1 / Preparation time: 5 minutes / Cooking time: 1 minute

1 tablespoon coconut flour

1 teaspoon cinnamon, divided

1 scoop vanilla protein powder

1 tablespoon and 1 teaspoon swerve sweetener, granulated

1/2 teaspoon baking powder

1/4 teaspoon vanilla extract, unsweetened

1/4 cup coconut cream

1/4 cup almond milk, unsweetened

- Take a medium heatproof bowl, grease with oil, then add flour, ½ teaspoon cinnamon, protein powder, 1 tablespoon swerve sweetener, baking powder and stir until well mixed.
- Slowly in coconut cream and milk until smooth batter comes together.
- Sprinkle with remaining cinnamon and sweetener and microwave for 1 minute or more until cake is cooked in the center.
- Serve straightaway.

Per Serving: Net Carbs: 7.6g; Calories: 302; Total Fat: 21.5g; Saturated Fat: 19.5g; Protein: 17.3g; Carbs: 9.8g; Fiber: 2.2g; Sugar: 5.2g

Percentage of Calories: Total Fat: 64%; Protein: 23%; Carbs: 13%;

Chocolate Avocado Ice Cream

Serves: 6 / Preparation time: 2 hours and 5 minutes / Cooking time: 10 minutes

2 medium avocado, pitted

1/3 cup swerve sweetener

1 1/2 teaspoon ground cinnamon

3/4 teaspoon chipotle powder

1 teaspoon vanilla extract, unsweetened

3 ounces dark chocolate, unsweetened

15-ounces coconut milk, full-fat and unsweetened

- Place a medium saucepan over medium heat, add espresso, sweetener, and milk and whisk well until sweetener is dissolved completely.
- Bring milk to simmer, then remove the pan from heat, stir in chocolate and let sit for 5 minutes.
- Whisk the mixture until smooth, stir in vanilla and pour the mixture in a food processor.
- Add remaining ingredients and pulse until smooth.
- Transfer mixture into a bowl and refrigerator for 2 hours until chilled.
- Then transfer mixture into ice cream maker and process until mixture reach to ice cream consistency.
- Serve straightaway or store in airtight container.

Per Serving: Net Carbs: 4.2g; Calories: 292.3; Total Fat: 25.7g; Saturated Fat: 13g; Protein: 4.2g; Carbs: 12.2g; Fiber: 8g; Sugar: 4g

Percentage of Calories: Total Fat: 79%; Protein: 4%; Carbs: 17%;

Coconut Fat Bombs

Serves: 18 / Preparation time: 5 minutes / Cooking time: 0 minutes

1/4 cup and 2 tablespoons shredded coconut

1/2 cup avocado oil

1/2 cup coconut butter, melted

12 drops stevia

- Place all the ingredients in a large bowl and stir until well mixed.
- Divide the mixture evenly in an ice cube tray and place in freezer until firm.
- Serve when ready.

Per Serving: Net Carbs: 1g; Calories: 85; Total Fat: 9g; Saturated Fat: 6g; Protein: 0g; Carbs: 1g; Fiber: 0g; Sugar: 0g

Percentage of Calories: Total Fat: 95%; Protein: 0%; Carbs: 5%;

Almond Fat Bombs

Serves: 10 / Preparation time: 5 minutes / Cooking time: 0 minutes

1/2 cup almond flour

1/8 teaspoon salt

16 drops stevia

1 teaspoon vanilla extract, unsweetened

1/2 teaspoon almond extract, unsweetened

1/2 cup avocado oil

20 slices of almonds

- Place all the ingredients in a large bowl and stir until well mixed.
- Divide the mixture evenly between 10 silicone molds and place in freezer until firm.
- Serve when ready.

Per Serving: Net Carbs: 1g; Calories: 125; Total Fat: 13g; Saturated Fat: 9g; Protein: 1g; Carbs: 1g; Fiber: 0g; Sugar: 0g

Percentage of Calories: Total Fat: 94%; Protein: 3%; Carbs: 3%;

Chocolate Peppermint Fat Bombs

Serves: 19 / Preparation time: 2 hours and 10 minutes / Cooking time: 0 minutes

Peppermint Filling:

12 drops of stevia

1 teaspoon peppermint extract, unsweetened

1/2 cup coconut butter, melted

1/2 cup avocado oil

Chocolate Coating:

20 drops of stevia

1 teaspoon vanilla extract, unsweetened

1/2 cup cacao powder, unsweetened

1/2 cup avocado oil

- Stir together all the ingredients for peppermint filling until mixed well.
- Spoon the mixture into ice cube tray and place in freezer for 2 hours or more until firm.
- Then stir together all the ingredients for chocolate coating until mixed well.
- When peppermint bombs are frozen, remove them from the tray and coat thoroughly with chocolate coating using a fork.
- Place chocolate coated peppermint bomb on a parchment sheet and freeze until hard.
- Serve straightaway.

Per Serving: Net Carbs: 1g; Calories: 125; Total Fat: 13g; Saturated Fat: 10g; Protein: 0g; Carbs: 2g; Fiber: 1g; Sugar: 0g

Percentage of Calories: Total Fat: 93%; Protein: 0%; Carbs: 6%;

Chocolate Fudge

Serves: 12 / Preparation time: 5 minutes / Cooking time: 0 minutes

1/2 cup cocoa powder, unsweetened

2 teaspoons erythritol sweetener

1/2 teaspoon vanilla extract, unsweetened

1 teaspoon almond extract, unsweetened

1/2 cup avocado oil

1/4 cup coconut milk, full-fat and unsweetened

- Place all the ingredients in a heatproof bowl and microwave for 1 minute or until melted.
- Stir well until sweetener is dissolved and then spoon the mixture into a bowl lined with plastic wrap.
- Place the bowl into the freezer until solid.
- Once frozen, pull out plastic wrap to take out fudge and slice into even pieces.
- Serve straightaway or store in freezer.

Per Serving: Net Carbs: 1g; Calories: 98; Total Fat: 10g; Saturated Fat: 9g; Protein: 0g; Carbs: 2g; Fiber: 1g; Sugar: 0g

Percentage of Calories: Total Fat: 92%; Protein: 0%; Carbs: 8%;

Chocolate Peppermint Chia Pudding

Serves: 6 / Preparation time: 3 hours and 5 minutes / Cooking time: 0 minutes

½ cup chia seeds

2 ¼ tablespoons cocoa powder, unsweetened

1 teaspoon sea salt

8 tablespoons swerve sweetener

1/2 teaspoon peppermint extract, unsweetened

1 tablespoon avocado oil

2 cups almond milk, full-fat unsweetened

¼ cup coconut milk, full-fat and unsweetened

- Place all the ingredients in a large bowl and stir until well mixed.
- Place the bowl in a refrigerator for 3 hours or more until chilled and smooth pudding comes together.
- Serve when ready.

Per Serving: Net Carbs: 2g; Calories: 117.3; Total Fat: 9.1g; Saturated Fat: 1.35g; Protein: 2.3g; Carbs: 6.4g; Fiber: 5.3g; Sugar: 0.2g

Percentage of Calories: Total Fat: 70%; Protein: 8%; Carbs: 22%;

Almond Cookies

Serves: 18 / Preparation time: 10 minutes / Cooking time: 25 minutes

4 teaspoons sliced almonds

1 cup almond flour

1 tablespoon flax meal

4 teaspoons erythritol sweetener

1 teaspoon baking powder

1/4 teaspoon salt

1 teaspoon vanilla extract, unsweetened

1/2 teaspoon almond extract, unsweetened

1/2 cup almond butter

1/2 cup almond milk, unsweetened

- Set oven to 350 degrees F and let preheat.
- In the meantime, stir together all the dry ingredients, from flour to salt, until mixed and then add almond butter.
- Whisk together extracts and milk and slowly mix into flour mixture until incorporated.
- Take a large baking sheet, line with parchment paper and then scoop prepared batter using an ice cream scoop.
- Press lightly to shape dough into cookies and then top each cookie with two almonds.
- Place the baking sheet into the oven and bake for 25 to 30 minutes or until golden brown.
- Serve straightaway.

Per Serving: Net Carbs: 2g; Calories: 87; Total Fat: 7g; Saturated Fat: 0g; Protein: 3g; Carbs: 3g; Fiber: 1g; Sugar: 0g

Percentage of Calories: Total Fat: 72%; Protein: 14%; Carbs: 14%;

Chocolate Almond Butter Cupcakes

Serves: 4 / Preparation time: 10 minutes / Cooking time: 30 minutes

2 tablespoons ground flax seeds

2 tablespoons cocoa powder, unsweetened

1/2 teaspoon baking powder

2 tablespoons swerve sweetener

1/4 cup almond butter, unsweetened

1/4 cup almond milk, unsweetened

For Frosting:

1 tablespoon almond butter, unsweetened

2 tablespoons vegan cream cheese

2 tablespoons almond milk, unsweetened and full-fat

- Set oven to 350 degrees F and let preheat.
- In the meantime, take 4 muffin cups, line with paper liners and set aside.
- Whisk together almond butter and milk in a large bowl until smooth.
- Then stir in flax seed and sweetener until combined and set aside.
- Stir together cocoa powder and baking powder with fork until combined and gradually stir into flaxseed mixture until smooth batter comes together.
- Divide the batter evenly between four muffin cups and then place them into the heated oven.
- Bake for 30 minutes or until firm and when done, cool for 20 minutes on wire rack and then take out muffins to cool completely.
- In the meantime, stir together all the ingredients of frosting, then top on muffins and serve.

Per Serving: Net Carbs: 3.5g; Calories: 272; Total Fat: 22g; Saturated Fat: 10g; Protein: 6.1g; Carbs: 12.5g; Fiber: 9g; Sugar: 2g

Percentage of Calories: Total Fat: 72%; Protein: 9%; Carbs: 18%;

Red Velvet Cupcakes

Serves: 4 / Preparation time: 10 minutes / Cooking time: 30 minutes

For Cupcakes:

2 tablespoons ground flax seed

2 tablespoons cocoa powder, unsweetened

2 tablespoons swerve sweetener

1 tablespoon beetroot powder

1/4 teaspoon baking soda

1/2 teaspoon baking powder

1 tablespoon apple cider vinegar

1/4 cup almond butter

1/4 cup coconut milk, unsweetened

For the Frosting:

5 drops of liquid stevia

1/4 cup coconut cream

1/4 cup vegan cream cheese

- Set oven to 350 degrees F and let preheat.
- In the meantime, line four muffin cups with paper liners and set aside.
- Whisk together vinegar, almond butter and coconut milk in a large bowl until smooth and then stir in flax seeds and sweetener.
- In another bowl, whisk together remaining ingredients for cupcake until combined and then gradually stir into milk mixture until smooth batter comes together.
- Divide the batter evenly between prepared muffin cups and then place into the oven.
- Bake muffin cups for 25 to 30 minutes or until firm.
- When done, cool muffin cups for 10 minutes on wire rack, then take out muffins and cool cupcakes completely.
- In the meantime, prepare frosting by whisking together all its ingredients until smooth.
- Top frosting over cooled cupcakes and serve.

Per Serving: Net Carbs: 4.7g; Calories: 230; Total Fat: 19g; Saturated Fat: 6g; Protein: 6g; Carbs: 9g; Fiber: 4.3g; Sugar: 0.6g

Percentage of Calories: Total Fat: 75%; Protein: 10%; Carbs: 15%;

REFERENCES AND RESOURCES

A Comprehensive Guide To The Vegan Ketogenic Diet | Ruled Me. (2018). Retrieved from https://www.ruled.me/comprehensive-guide-vegan-ketogenic-diet/

Craig, W. (2009). Health effects of vegan diets. *The American Journal Of Clinical Nutrition*, *89*(5), 1627S-1633S. doi: 10.3945/ajcn.2009.26736n

Easy Guide to the Vegan Ketogenic Diet for 2018 | Get Started!. Retrieved from http://ketomotive.com/vegan-ketogenic-diet/

Iacovides, S., & Meiring, R. (2018). The effect of a ketogenic diet versus a high-carbohydrate, low-fat diet on sleep, cognition, thyroid function, and cardiovascular health independent of weight loss: study protocol for a randomized controlled trial. *Trials*, *19*(1). doi: 10.1186/s13063-018-2462-5

Jami Cooley, C. (2018). Keto Diet: The Fat-Burning Health Benefits of Ketogenic Diet Foods. Retrieved from https://universityhealthnews.com/daily/nutrition/keto-diet-health-benefits-of-ketogenic-diet/

Johnstone, A., Horgan, G., Murison, S., Bremner, D., & Lobley, G. (2008). Effects of a high-protein ketogenic diet on hunger, appetite, and weight loss in obese men feeding ad libitum. *The American Journal Of Clinical Nutrition*, *87*(1), 44-55. doi: 10.1093/ajcn/87.1.44

Le, L., & Sabaté, J. (2014). Beyond Meatless, the Health Effects of Vegan Diets: Findings from the Adventist Cohorts. *Nutrients*, *6*(6), 2131-2147. doi: 10.3390/nu6062131

Nordqvist, C. (2018). Vegan diet: Health benefits, risks, and meal tips. Retrieved from https://www.medicalnewstoday.com/articles/149636.php?sr

Paoli, A., Bosco, G., Camporesi, E., & Mangar, D. (2015). Ketosis, ketogenic diet and food intake control: a complex relationship. *Frontiers In Psychology*, *6*. doi: 10.3389/fpsyg.2015.00027

Pierre-Louis, K. (2017). Vegetarian and vegan diets aren't necessarily more healthy. Retrieved from https://www.popsci.com/vegetarian-vegan-not-always-healthy#page-2

Railton, D. (2018). Nutrition 2018: New data confirm health benefits of plant-based diet. Retrieved from https://www.medicalnewstoday.com/articles/322072.php

Rizzo, G., Laganà, A., Rapisarda, A., La Ferrera, G., Buscema, M., & Rossetti, P. et al. (2016). Vitamin B12 among Vegetarians: Status, Assessment and Supplementation. *Nutrients*, *8*(12), 767. doi: 10.3390/nu8120767

Rogerson, D. (2017). Vegan diets: practical advice for athletes and exercisers. *Journal Of The International Society Of Sports Nutrition*, *14*(1). doi: 10.1186/s12970-017-0192-9Rozenberg, S., Body,

J., Bruyère, O., Bergmann, P., Brandi, M., & Cooper, C. et al. (2015). Effects of Dairy Products Consumption on Health: Benefits and Beliefs—A Commentary from the Belgian Bone Club and the European Society for Clinical and Economic Aspects of Osteoporosis, Osteoarthritis and Musculoskeletal Diseases. *Calcified Tissue International*, *98*(1), 1-17. doi: 10.1007/s00223-015-0062-x

Sinha, R., Cross, A., Graubard, B., Leitzmann, M., & Schatzkin, A. (2009). Meat Intake and Mortality. *Archives Of Internal Medicine*, *169*(6), 562. doi: 10.1001/archinternmed.2009.6

Slavin, J., & Lloyd, B. (2012). Health Benefits of Fruits and Vegetables. *Advances In Nutrition*, *3*(4), 506-516. doi: 10.3945/an.112.002154

Tuso, P. (2013). Nutritional Update for Physicians: Plant-Based Diets. *The Permanente Journal*, *17*(2), 61-66. doi: 10.7812/tpp/12-085

Vegan Ketogenic Diet: Everything You Need To Know To Get Started. Retrieved from https://www.wellnessgeeky.com/vegan-ketogenic-diet/

Wolk, A. (2016). Potential health hazards of eating red meat. *Journal Of Internal Medicine*, *281*(2), 106-122. doi: 10.1111/joim.12543

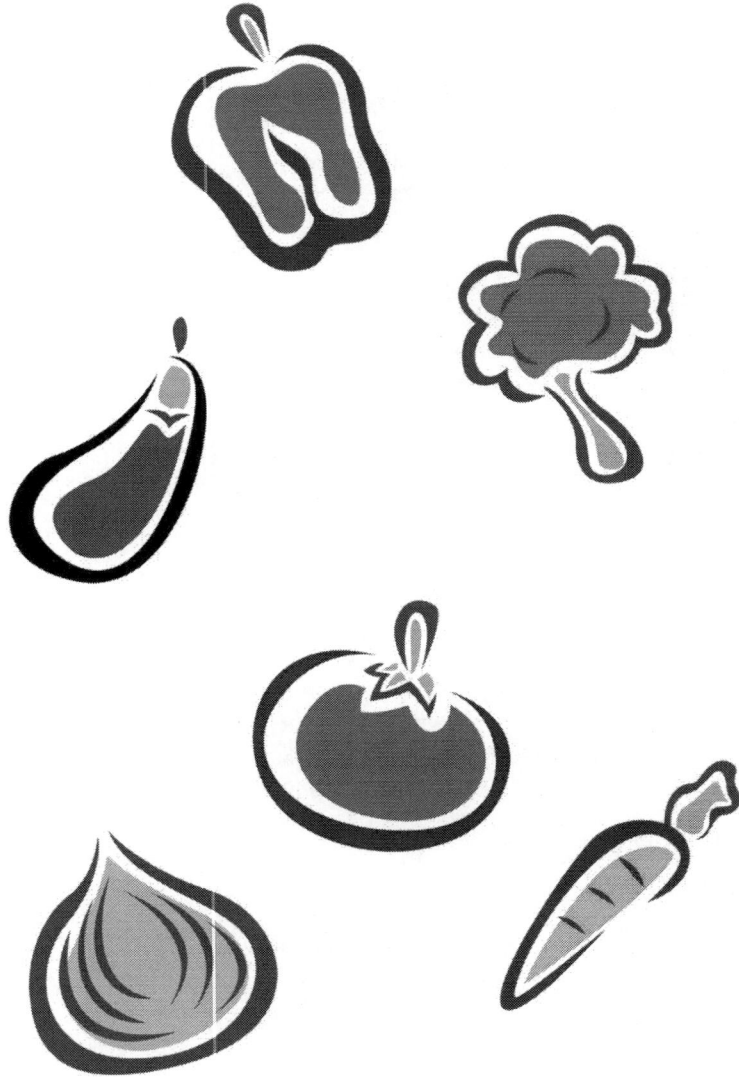

THE "DIRTY DOZEN" AND "CLEAN 15"

Every year, the Environmental Working Group releases a list of the produce with the most pesticide residue (Dirty Dozen) and a list of the ones with the least **chance of having residue (Clean 15). It's based on analysis from the U.S.** Department of Agriculture Pesticide Data Program report.

The Environmental Working Group found that 70% of the 48 types of produce tested had residues of at least one type of pesticide. In total there were 178 different pesticides and pesticide breakdown products. This residue can stay on veggies and fruit even after they are washed and peeled. All pesticides are toxic to humans and consuming them can cause damage to the nervous system, reproductive system, cancer, a weakened immune system, and more. Women who are pregnant can expose their unborn children to toxins through their diet, and continued exposure to pesticides can affect their development.

This info can help you choose the best fruits and veggies, as well as which ones you should always try to buy organic.

The Dirty Dozen

- Strawberries
- Spinach
- Nectarines
- Apples
- Peaches
- Celery
- Grapes
- Pears
- Cherries
- Tomatoes
- Sweet bell peppers
- Potatoes

The Clean 15

- Sweet corn
- Avocados
- Pineapples
- Cabbage
- Onions
- Frozen sweet peas
- Papayas
- Asparagus
- Mangoes
- Eggplant
- Honeydew
- Kiwi
- Cantaloupe
- Cauliflower
- Grapefruit

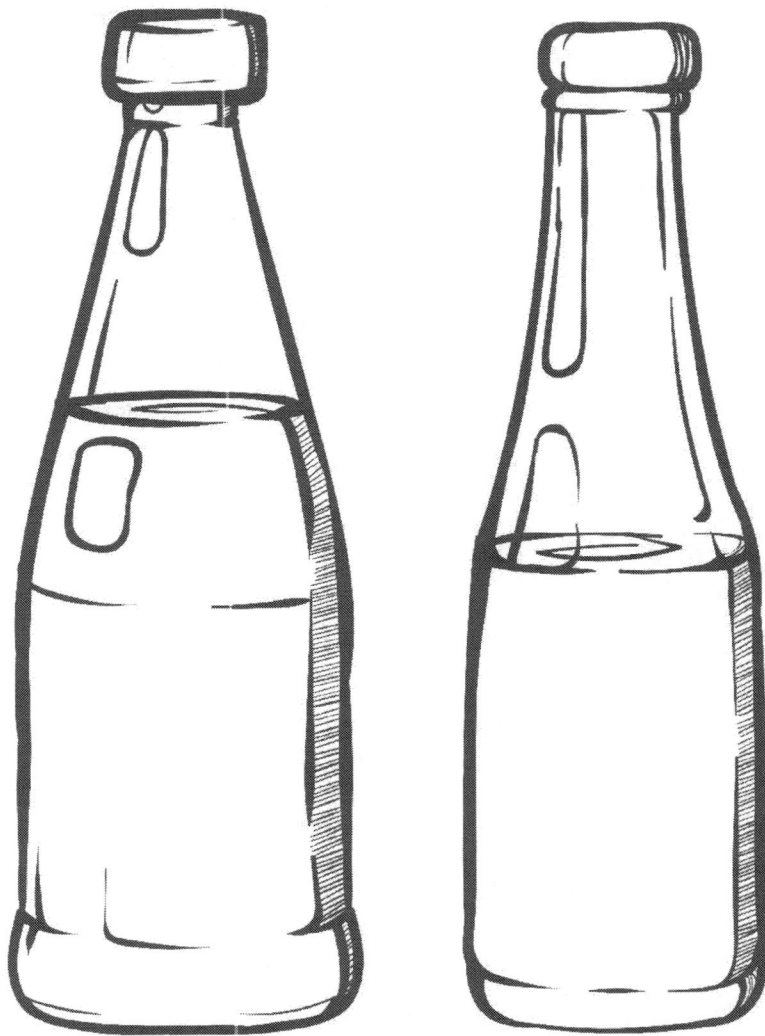

MEASUREMENT CONVERSION TABLES

VOLUME EQUIVALENTS (DRY)

US Standard	Metric (Approx.)
¼ teaspoon	1 ml
½ teaspoon	2 ml
1 teaspoon	5 ml
1 tablespoon	15 ml
¼ cup	59 ml
½ cup	118 ml
1 cup	235 ml

WEIGHT EQUIVALENTS

US Standard	Metric (Approx.)
½ ounce	15 g
1 ounce	30 g
2 ounces	60 g
4 ounces	115 g
8 ounces	225 g
12 ounces	340 g
16 oz or 1 lb	455 g

VOLUME EQUIVALENTS (LIQUID)

US Standard	US Standard (ounces)	Metric (Approx.)
2 tablespoons	1 fl oz	30 ml
¼ cup	2 fl oz	60 ml
½ cup	4 fl oz	120 ml
1 cup	8 fl oz	240 ml
1 ½ cups	12 fl oz	355 ml
2 cups or 1 pint	16 fl oz	475 ml
4 cups or 1 quart	32 fl oz	1 L
1 gallon	128 fl oz	4 L

OVEN TEMPERATURES

Fahrenheit (F)	Celsius (C) (Approx)
250°F	120°C
300°F	150°C
325°F	165°C
350°F	180°C
375°F	190°C
400°F	200°C
425°F	220°C
450°F	230°C

INDEX

A

Almond Avocado Pudding, 128
Almond Cookies, 138
Almond Fat Bombs, 134
Avocado Arugula Salad, 56
Avocado Chocolate Mousse, 130

B

Bagels, 36
Balsamic Glazed Mushrooms, 98
Basil Pesto Zucchini Noodles, 80
Berries Smoothie, 38
Bibimbap, 91
Broccoli Fried Rice, 101

C

Caesar Salad, 60
Cauliflower and Greens Smoothie Bowl, 31
Cauliflower Fried Rice, 111
Cauliflower Pizza Crust, 118
Cauliflower Rice Pilaf, 119
Cauliflower Tofu Tacos, 108
Chocolate Almond Butter Cupcakes, 139
Chocolate Avocado Ice Cream, 132
Chocolate Fondue, 127
Chocolate Fudge, 136
Chocolate Peppermint Chia Pudding, 137
Chocolate Peppermint Fat Bombs, 135
Cinnamon Chocolate Smoothie, 33
Cinnamon Roll Mug Cake, 131
Coconut Bacon, 86
Coconut Dulce De Leche, 126
Coconut Fat Bombs, 133
Coconut Porridge, 43
Crack Slaw, 63
Crackers, 85
Cream of Mushroom Soup, 52
Creamy Broccoli Soup, 68
Cucumber Salad, 66
Curried Tofu Scramble, 30
Curry Noodle Bowls, 61

D

Deviled Avocado, 78
Doughnuts, 45

E

Egg Roll Bowl, 65

F

Falafel, 93
Flaxseed Waffles, 34
Fried Tempeh, 72
Fudge Oats, 28

G

Garlic Aioli, 82
Ginger Coleslaw, 59
Gingerbread Muffins, 46
Green Coffee Shake, 35
Green Soup, 55
Guacamole, 84

H

Halloumi Salad, 64
Hemp Heart Porridge, 37
Hemp Seed Lettuce Wraps, 120

K

Kale & Crispy Coconut Tempeh, 113
Kale and Spinach Soup, 69
Kelp Noodles with Avocado Pesto, 92

L

Lemon Pancakes, 29

M

Maple Oatmeal, 32
Maple Oatmeal Breakfast Bites, 42
Mashed Garlic Cauliflower, 97
Mint Matcha Fat Bombs, 76
Mozzarella Sticks, 73

O

Omelet, 44

P

Parmesan Fried Eggplant, 79
Peanut Shirataki noodles, 104
Portobello Mushroom "Tacos", 117

R

Red Curry Cauliflower Soup, 51

Red Velvet Cupcakes, 140
Roasted Bok Choy, 83
Roasted Cabbage with Lemon, 95
Roasted Cauliflower Steaks, 74
Roasted Eggplant, 96
Roasted Lemon Vegetables, 115
Roasted Radishes, 75
Roasted Red Pepper Soup, 53

S

Sage and Cheddar Waffles, 41
Shirataki Noodles with Almond Butter Sauce, 110
Sloppy Joes, 90
Spinach and Artichoke Soup, 67
Spinach and Tofu Scramble, 47
Spinach Artichoke Pizza, 122
Strawberry Chia Pudding, 129
Stuffed Avocado, 40
Superfood Keto, 54

T

Thai Soup, 50

Toasted Coconut Cashews, 77
Tofu & Cauliflower Rice, 103
Tofu and Shirataki Noodle, 94
Tofu in Purgatory, 112
Tomato Mushroom Spaghetti Squash, 58
Triple Green Kale Salad, 57

W

Walnut Chili, 121
Whole Roasted Cauliflower, 100

Z

Zucchini Cakes, 81
Zucchini Cauliflower Fritters, 39
Zucchini Lasagna, 114
Zucchini Noodles with Avocado Sauce, 102
Zucchini Noodles with Hemp Pesto, 99
Zucchini Pasta, 116
Zucchini Salad, 62
Zucchini Tomato Pesto, 109

30 DAY MEAL PLAN

QTY	BREAKFAST	LUNCH	DINNER
1	Berries Smoothie 38	Broccoli Fried Rice 101	Roasted Lemon Vegetables 115
2	Fudge Oats 28	Bibimbap 91	Walnut Chili 121
3	Maple Oatmeal Breakfast Bites 42	Tofu and Shirataki Noodle 94	Cauliflower Fried Rice 111
4	Flaxseed Waffles 34	Zucchini Noodles with Hemp Pesto 99	Kale & Crispy Coconut Tempeh 113
5	Stuffed Avocado 40	Peanut Shirataki noodles 104	Cauliflower Tofu Tacos 108
6	Cauliflower and Greens Smoothie Bowl 31	Sloppy Joes 90	Cauliflower Rice Pilaf 119
7	Lemon Pancakes 29	Roasted Eggplant 96	Zucchini Lasagna 114
8	Sage and Cheddar Waffles 41	Zucchini Noodles with Avocado Sauce 102	Zucchini Tomato Pesto 109
9	Cinnamon Chocolate Smoothie 33	Mashed Garlic Cauliflower 97	Portobello Mushroom "Tacos" 117
10	Zucchini Cauliflower Fritters 39	Kelp Noodles with Avocado Pesto 92	Shirataki Noodles with Almond Butter Sauce 110
11	Maple Oatmeal 32	Whole Roasted Cauliflower 100	Zucchini Pasta 116
12	Doughnuts 45	Balsamic Glazed Mushrooms 98	Hemp Seed Lettuce Wraps 120
13	Hemp Heart Porridge 37	Falafel 93	Tofu in Purgatory 112
14	Lemon Pancakes 29	Tofu & Cauliflower Rice 103	Cauliflower Pizza Crust 118
15	Flaxseed Waffles 34	Roasted Cabbage with Lemon 95	Spinach Artichoke Pizza 122

16	Spinach and Tofu Scramble 47	Broccoli Fried Rice 101	Cauliflower Pizza Crust 118
17	Bagels 36	Roasted Eggplant 96	Zucchini Lasagna 114
18	Omelet 44	Bibimbap 91	Hemp Seed Lettuce Wraps 120
19	Green Coffee Shake 35	Peanut Shirataki noodles 104	Roasted Lemon Vegetables 115
20	Maple Oatmeal Breakfast Bites 42	Tofu and Shirataki Noodle 94	Kale & Crispy Coconut Tempeh 113
21	Cinnamon Chocolate Smoothie 33	Sloppy Joes 90	Cauliflower Rice Pilaf 119
22	Berries Smoothie 38	Zucchini Noodles with Avocado Sauce 102	Tofu in Purgatory 112
23	Spinach and Tofu Scramble 47	Roasted Cabbage with Lemon 95	Spinach Artichoke Pizza 122
24	Coconut Porridge 43	Mashed Garlic Cauliflower 97	Zucchini Tomato Pesto 109
25	Fudge Oats 28	Kelp Noodles with Avocado Pesto 92	Cauliflower Tofu Tacos 108
26	Gingerbread Muffins 46	Balsamic Glazed Mushrooms 98	Portobello Mushroom "Tacos" 117
27	Sage and Cheddar Waffles 41	Whole Roasted Cauliflower 100	Cauliflower Fried Rice 111
28	Green Coffee Shake 35	Bibimbap 91	Zucchini Pasta 116
29	Doughnuts 45	Zucchini Noodles with Hemp Pesto 99	Walnut Chili 121
30	Cauliflower and Greens Smoothie Bowl 31	Falafel 93	Shirataki Noodles with Almond Butter Sauce 110